Orthopaedic splint and appliances

By
Joan M. Kennedy
M.C.S.P., O.N.C.
Formerly Lecturer in Practical Orthopaedics
Superintendent Orthopaedic After-Care Sister
Nuffield Orthopaedic Centre, Oxford

With a foreword by
Professor R. B. Duthie
Nuffield Professor of Orthopaedic Surgery
University of Oxford

BAILLIÈRE TINDALL LONDON

Baillière Tindall
7 & 8 Henrietta Street, London WC2E 8QE

Cassell & Collier Macmillan Publishers Limited, London
35 Red Lion Square, London WC1R 4SG
Sydney, Auckland, Toronto, Johannesburg

The Macmillan Publishing Co. Inc.
New York

© 1974 Baillière Tindall

All rights reserved. No part of this publication may be
reproduced, stored in a retrieval system, or transmitted,
in any form or by any means, electronic, mechanical,
photocopying, recording or otherwise, without the prior
permission of Baillière Tindall

First published 1974

ISBN 0 7020 0469 3

Published in the United States of America by
the Williams & Wilkins Company, Baltimore

Printed in Great Britain by
The Whitefriars Press Ltd, London and Tonbridge

Foreword

The traditional orthopaedic workshop is now shaking itself free from the shackles of antiquity and of its image being made up of brace makers. This has been brought about by the coming of newer materials and by the work of such people as the author of this book, Miss Joan Kennedy. She has had the unique position of being trained both as an orthopaedic nurse as well as a physiotherapist and has led, for many years, a Department of After-Care Sisters. I cannot think of anyone better to have produced such a textbook on this subject.

Unfortunately at the present time this subject is being poorly taught to both nurses and doctors in training but this book with its extensive and well illustrated coverage should provide a most valuable text and reference for everyone working in this field. Considering that the national bill to the National Health Service for surgical appliances and orthotics, etc., is over £9 million, there is no excuse for anyone having the responsibility of prescribing, fitting and ensuring function of these therapeutic modalities, not to have this knowledge. It is surprising how little advance has been made in the design and function of orthopaedic splints and appliances. Therefore I recommend this book most highly to all those engaged in orthotic care of patients, to those who teach and, of course, to all in training.

November 1973   R. B. DUTHIE

Preface

In writing this book on orthopaedic splints and appliances I have tried to consider the needs of the orthopaedic nurse, physiotherapist, after-care sisters, doctors, and medical students when confronted with the patient and the consequent splint problem. I have therefore included a comprehensive section on plaster work and plaster casts. Plaster splints are the cheapest and most adaptable of splints, but they need to be carefully made. Plaster casts are essential for the measurements of moulded leather and many plastic splints.

I have included several of the synthetic materials in general use with their advantages and disadvantages. I have also given a selection of splints for individual conditions, as not all patients tolerate the same splint. Measurements and procedures are given where practicable for each splint. The subject of prosthesis and the making and fitting of the artificial limb has been excluded in so much as this highly technical field is already catered for.

I hope, therefore, that this book will enable the student to understand the functions of the splints and appliances, and that the correct splinting of difficult conditions will prove less of a challenge.

I am much indebted to my many colleagues for their help and encouragement, especially Mr J. C. Scott, F.R.C.S., for his wise advice, Mr R. Emanuel for his photography, Mrs D. Wilkins for typing the manuscript, and Mr F. W. Weston, Superintendent of The Nuffield Orthopaedic Workshops, for his help and co-operation, and producing splints when required. I should also like to thank my fellow after-care sisters for their help in allowing their patients to be photographed. I am also indebted to Professor R. B. Duthie, The Nuffield Professor of Orthopaedic Surgery, University of Oxford, for having the manuscript read in his department. I cannot finish this foreword without acknowledging the willing help I have had from many orthopaedic centres in this country. I hope they will find the book useful.

Acknowledgments

I would like to thank the following individuals for allowing me to use illustrations: Mr M. P. McCormack (Figs 103 and 142), Mr M. H. M. Harrison (Fig. 82), Mrs B. Hughes (Figs 106, 134 and 143), Mr John P. O'Brien (Fig. 120), Mr J. Rowland Hughes (Fig. 145), Mr G. K. Rose (Fig. 73), Mr D. L. Savill (Figs 46 to 49), Messrs W. J. Sharrard and Herzog (Fig. 75), and Mr W. H. Tuck (Fig. 25). I also acknowledge the help of the following firms for the use of their information and photographs: S. H. Camp & Co. Ltd, Johnson & Johnson, Nottingham Handcraft Co. Ltd, Pryor & Howard, Remploy Ltd, Smith & Nephew Ltd, Spencer Surgical Supplies, and Zimmer Ltd.

November 1973   JOAN M. KENNEDY

Contents

	Foreword	iii
	Preface	v
	Introductory note	viii
1	Plaster of Paris	1
2	Moulded leather splints	32
3	Splints made from synthetic materials	34
4	Hand and finger splints	48
5	Wrist splints	65
6	Elbow splints	67
7	Shoulder splints	72
8	Calipers	75
9	Spina bifida cystica	94
10	Perthe's disease	103
11	Congenital dislocated hip	109
12	Knee splints	114
13	Below-knee irons	119
14	Congenital foot deformity splints	128
15	Insoles and shoe adaptations	137
16	Spinal braces	151
17	Collars	164
18	Surgical belts and corsets	168
19	Crutches and walking aids	174
20	Bed appliances	183
	Index	197

INTRODUCTORY NOTE

Splints and appliances can be used to help the patient in several different ways. A splint may take the place of a paralysed muscle, or diseased joint—or it may assist a weak muscle or joint. In some cases, splints may help to relieve a joint of some of the body weight, or can be designed to protect a vulnerable joint. Bed splints are usually designed to rest the limbs in the optimum position of use and, of course, they are used for the relief of pain. Appliances can also be designed to correct deformities and to maintain a correction. Thought must, however, be given to the cosmetic appearance, weight and durability of the splint; and use made of the wide choice of materials available. Anatomical knowledge is a great help in the measuring, fitting and application of splints. A sympathetic approach to the patient and the parent is always necessary.

1

Plaster of Paris

Plaster of Paris is the cheapest form of splinting, and can also be one of the most comfortable if properly applied. It can be applied to any part of the body in any climatic conditions and in any building, provided that water and plaster of Paris bandages are available. Plaster is used for immobilization of joints and limbs after trauma and surgery, in cases of sepsis, for correcting deformities, maintaining correction, and as night splints and removable day splints. Plaster of Paris also forms an important part in the measuring of many splints and appliances, it is used for taking casts of the appropriate joints and limbs.

COMPOSITION OF PLASTER OF PARIS

The commercial types of plaster are now generally used, as they are easy to handle. Each bandage is individually wrapped in greaseproof paper and has a central plastic core, they keep well and storage is facilitated. A dry atmosphere is, however, essential.

Plaster of Paris in its free state is calcium sulphate dihydrate ($2CaSO_4.H_2O$). Gypsum is a fine grained white crystalline dihydrate with 21 per cent by weight of water. The plaster is formed by roasting crushed gypsum at 120° to 130°C so that it contains 6 per cent weight of water of crystallization.

SETTING OF PLASTERS

When plaster of Paris is added to water at room temperature a reaction takes place in two stages:

(1) The plaster takes up the water, sets in 4 to 5 min, but has at this stage only 35 to 50 per cent of ultimate strength.
(2) Excess water gradually evaporates, over several hours or even days, when the ultimate strength is obtained.

The process of setting is accompanied by expansion due to production of heat, this disappears when the cast loses warmth, this generally takes about 45 min. It is cold and clammy until really dry.

PLASTER OF PARIS BANDAGES

These bandages fall into two categories: (1) the gypsum bandage, and (2) the low plaster loss bandage.

The Gypsum Bandage

Gypsum bandages are made of good quality gauze of 28 to 32 threads per inch. The plaster is bound to the gauze by a dry bonder such as methyl cellulose which prevents it falling out of the bandage. Gypsum bandages are most suitable for taking plaster casts.

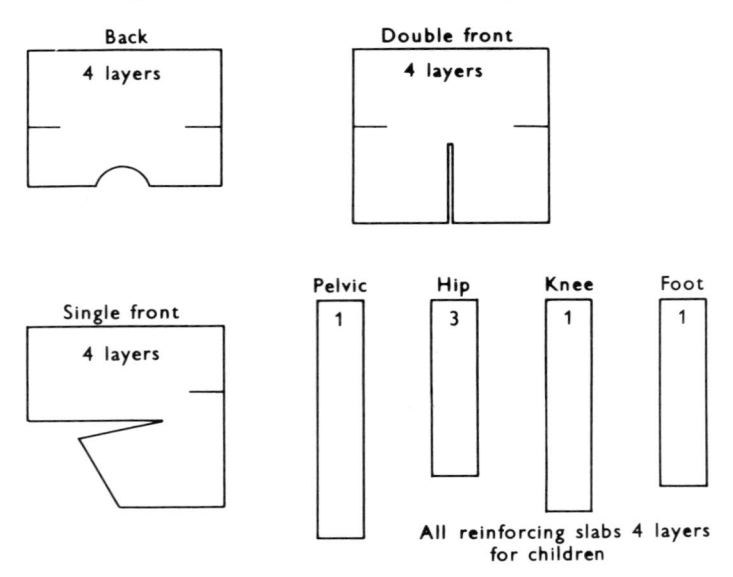

Back — 4 layers
Double front — 4 layers
Single front — 4 layers
Pelvic 1
Hip 3
Knee 1
Foot 1

All reinforcing slabs 4 layers for children

Fig. 1. Hip spica patterns.

Low Plaster Loss Bandages

Low plaster loss bandages have the addition of a wet binder, polyvinyl acetate, which leaves less residue in the bucket. The bandages are stronger, and fewer are needed. They are, however, less easy to handle and require more rubbing in at the setting stage. They are most suitable for plasters with a certain amount of strain to be exerted on them, such as those used for walking and jackets.

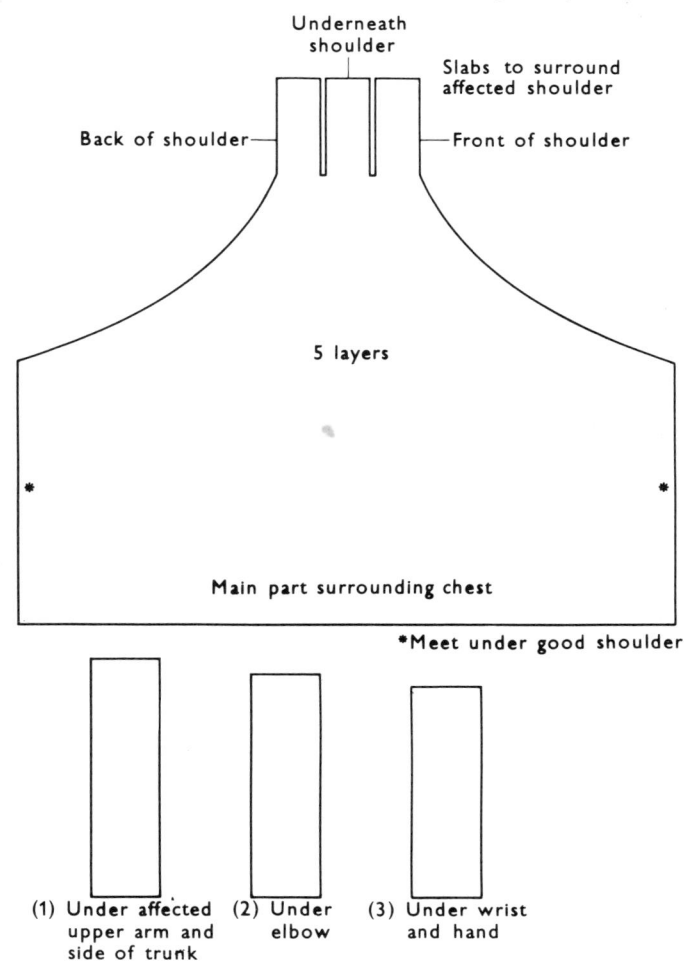

Underneath shoulder

Slabs to surround affected shoulder

Back of shoulder

Front of shoulder

5 layers

Main part surrounding chest

*Meet under good shoulder

(1) Under affected upper arm and side of trunk
(2) Under elbow
(3) Under wrist and hand

Fig. 2. Shoulder spica pattern.

The constant immersion time of a plaster bandage in water is 5 to 10 s, and the setting time is about 4 to 10 min (due to the inclusion of an accelerator, potassium sulphate).

Dry slabs for reinforcement can be prepared beforehand. A knowledge of the patterns that can be cut out of the wide rolls of Gypsona is useful. These rolls are made in widths of 18, 24 and 36 in. (40, 60 and 70 cm) (Figs 1 to 4).

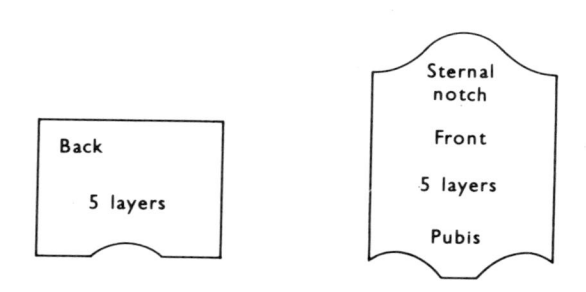

Fig. 3. High jacket pattern.

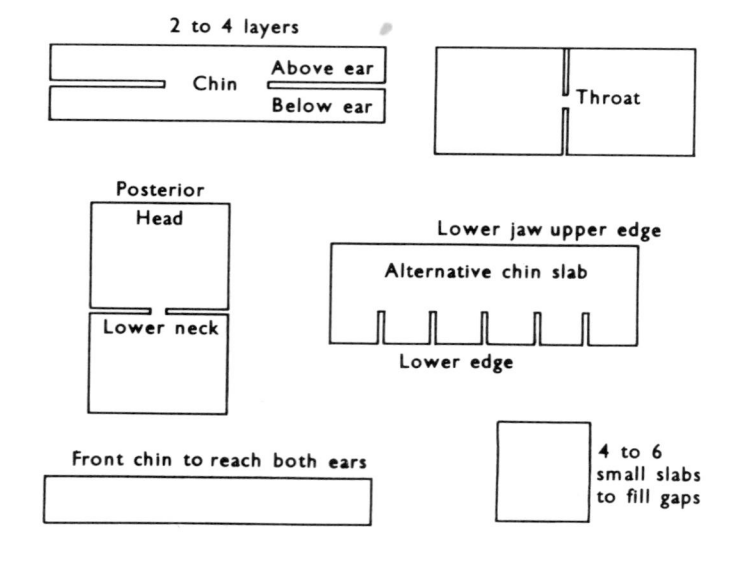

Fig. 4. Collar patterns.

HOME MADE PLASTER OF PARIS BANDAGES

Home made plaster of Paris bandages may be made on the spot. Book muslin, superfine plaster of Paris and a wide wooden table are all the materials required.

Method. The muslin is torn into strips either 4 yd x 6 in. or 3 yd x 4 in. These strips are rolled into bandages and the three outer threads removed from either end of the bandage. The plaster is then evenly impregnated into the prepared strips of muslin. These are unwound before rubbing the plaster evenly on the muslin, and the bandages are carefully rolled at the same time as the plaster is rubbed in. They need to be handled with care and stored in a dry place. Never handle with a wet hand or hard patches will appear. When the bandage is immersed in a bucket of warm water it will need to be squeezed in a concertina fashion before being used.

TECHNIQUE OF PLASTERING

Application of plaster should always be carefully done, as this makes all the difference to the comfort of the patient.

Before beginning a plaster the operator should know the patient's disability and consequently the type of plaster and padding required. The position of the joint is most important.

PADDING

Skin Tight Plasters

These plasters are used for some types of fractures, and should be glove fitting, and perfectly applied.

Stockinette and Felt

Felt strips or pads are placed over the stockinette, the bony points and sometimes at the edges of the plasters. This combination gives a well-fitting plaster.

Stretched Felt

White felt, $\frac{1}{4}$ in. (6 mm) thick, can be stretched round the trunk in the case of the application of a hip spica, or can be used for padding a jacket on a very thin patient. Care should be taken to see that the felt is applied with the stretch encircling the trunk. It is then sewn together at the junction of the limits of the felt.

Wool Padding

Plaster wool in the form of bandages is applied to limbs where swelling of a limb is expected, or where correction of deformity is to be carried out. It is, therefore, always used for post-operative plasters. Particular attention must be paid to the amount of padding required when plasters are being applied to correct deformities, for example in spastic cases, where there will be pressure in one or two points, or when applying a Risser type jacket, where considerable pressure is exerted over the maximum convexity of a curve during correction.

APPLICATION OF PLASTER OF PARIS

Materials required. A trolley should be laid out equipped with:

(1) An assortment of 2-, 4-, 6- and 8-in. (5-, 10-, 15- and 20-cm) Gypsona bandages.
(2) An assortment of 3- and 4-in. (7·5- and 10-cm) wool bandages.
(3) A selection of sharp cobblers knives.
(4) One pair of Elastoplast scissors.
(5) Indelible pencil.

A bucket of warm water, preferably resting in a bucket stand, must be available; a deep bowl may suffice, but there should be sufficient water to well cover the bandages. Some protective sheets, usually polythene sheeting, or even newspapers are helpful.

Application

(1) Apply necessary padding to the limb.
(2) The limb should be held in the correct position.
(3) Soak the plaster bandage; this is done by removing the outer

wrapping, freeing the end of the bandage and immersing it in the bucket of water. When the air bubbles have all escaped, gently lift the bandage out of the water, squeeze carefully towards the centre of the bandage and hold the bandage in one hand with the free end in the opposite hand.

(4) Roll the bandage gently and evenly around the limb, overlapping half the previous turn. Never let the bandage leave the limb except when making a pleat to fit a contour. Mould the plaster carefully at the same time as it is being applied. Reinforce all joints with reinforcing slabs. Rub the plaster well just as it is setting, this will ensure a strong cast and gives it a smooth surface. There should be no movement of the limb during application. If the position is altered during setting time, 70 per cent of the ultimate strength is lost. The plaster should be of a even thickness throughout to eliminate weak areas. A properly applied and reinforced plaster, with suitable slabs, does not need to be a heavy or thick one.

DRYING A PLASTER

All recently applied plasters should rest on a soft surface, such as a pillow covered with a rough towel or paper tissues. They should always be exposed to warm air for 24 to 36 hr. Walking plasters should be non-weight bearing for 2 to 3 days. Plaster jackets in particular should be uncovered day and night for at least 24 hr. Plasters applied after trauma should be elevated to prevent swelling of the extremities. The slabs for inclusion in a plaster can be prepared beforehand. This also applies to patterns for the larger plasters. These are cut out of a rolls of Gypsona which are available in widths of 18, 24 and 36 in. (see Figs 1 to 4).

TYPES OF PLASTER

The two most common plasters are the wrist plaster and the below-knee walking plaster.

Wrist Plaster or Colles Type

A wrist or Colles type plaster (Fig. 5) extends from below the elbow to the lower palmar crease, thus allowing full movement at the

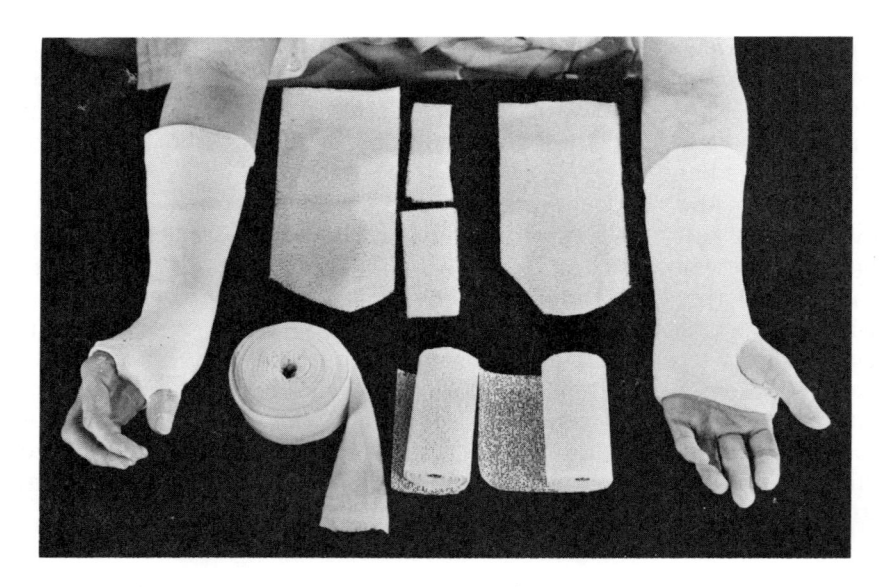

Fig. 5. Photograph showing a Colles plaster (right, note freedom of the thumb and fingers), and a scaphoid plaster (left, note the position of the thumb). In the centre are shown patterns, bandages and stockinette.

elbow and the fingers, at the same time allowing full opposition of the thumb. The wrist should be immobilized in about 30 degrees of extension.

Scaphoid Plaster

This is a forearm plaster with the thumb included. The thumb is immobilized in flexion, abduction and opposition, and the plaster extends to the interphalangeal joint, allowing flexion of the terminal phalanx.

Both the above plasters should have a palmar reinforcement or a slab, 4 in. (10 cm) wide and be made of four layers. The scaphoid plaster also needs two narrow strips for reinforcing the thumb.

The Elbow

This joint is not so frequently immobilized in plaster. If plaster is to be used, the elbow is flexed at right angles. Stockinette or wool padding is used, but special care must be taken to pad the elbow and wrist joint, two prominent bony points.

Hanging Plaster

The weight of the arm combined with a plaster that extends from well over the shoulder, including the point of the elbow up to the fracture site, is used after reduction of some types of fractured

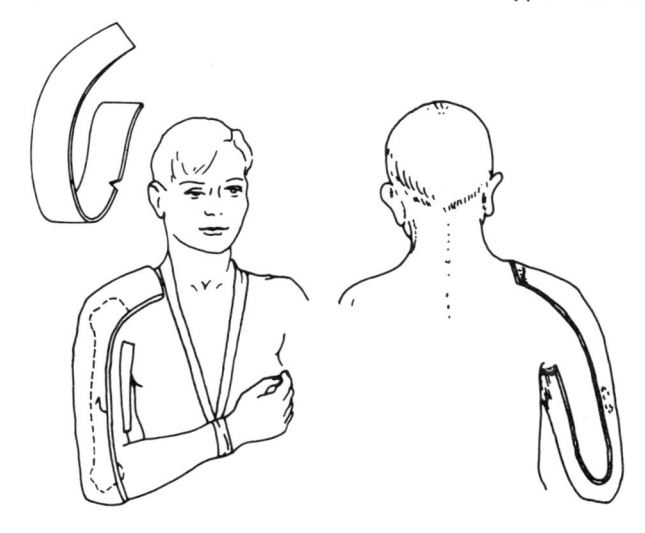

Fig. 6. Hanging plaster.

humerus. A collar and cuff is used to support the forearm. A long U-shaped plaster slab is made to cover the upper arm, and can be fixed by a gauze or Kling bandage. Alternatively the slab may be held in position with a plaster bandage. When using a cotton bandage to hold a plaster slab in position, it should always be immersed in water first to avoid shrinkage of the cotton bandage.

Shoulder Spica

The only way of really immobilizing a shoulder joint is by means of a thoracobrachial or shoulder spica. This comprises a large plaster and involves covering the affected arm and the trunk including the iliac crests. The trunk is vested with the addition of felt strips round the pelvis and over the affected shoulder. The arm is covered with plaster wool and felt pads cover the elbow and wrist joints. The arm is supported in 60 to 90 degrees of abduction, some flexion and internal rotation.

The shoulder spica pattern should be cut out from a 36-in. roll of Gypsona, and the subsidiary slabs prepared. The plaster is then applied, especial care being taken at the junction of the arm with the trunk. The plaster takes the weight of the arm. It should not be necessary to use a strut connecting the under surface of the elbow with the side of the trunk (Fig. 2).

Plaster Collars

A plaster collar is a test of the technique of the plasterer. The position of the head is all important, extension should be such that the patient is looking straight ahead, not upwards or downwards. Rotation and side flexion should be neutral.

Technique. The patient's lower occiput, chin and front of the neck to 5 in. (12·5 cm) below the sternal notch, and similar level posteriorly, should be covered in well-fitting sewn stretched felt (Fig. 7). A number of plaster slabs should be prepared beforehand. Three layers for each slab is sufficient. The slabs should be applied first and then fixed in position by not more than two 4-in. (10-cm) Gypsona bandages (Fig. 4). The edges of the plaster being carefully

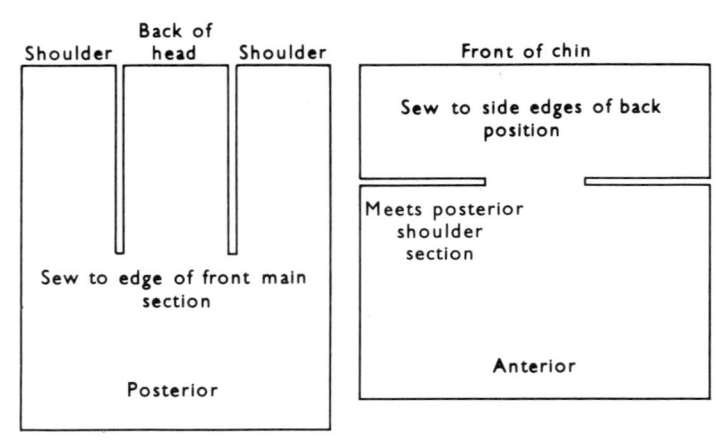

Fig. 7. Suggested patterns for felt application.

trimmed at the end, and the felt cut flush with the plaster. It is important to leave the ears free and to have at least a ½-in. (1-cm) shelf in *front* of the chin. All head movements should be restricted if the plaster is carefully applied. A similar method is used for a cast of the neck, but the neck is oiled instead of felted.

Plaster Jackets

Patients who have been in bed for several weeks and are consequently unable to stand may have the jacket applied while lying in the supine position supported on a metal framework. This framework is sometimes known as a Goldthwaite table and is designed so that the patient is supported under the shoulders, pelvis, knees and ankles by means of slings and padded bars, thus leaving the trunk free. Patients who are able to stand, and this applies to the many out-patients with low back pain, can have their jackets applied without any apparatus, providing their arms are supported on convenient rests (such as the backs of two chairs).

Ideally, if a Sayers apparatus is available the patient can stand on a raised platform and hold on to the two upright bars on either side (Fig. 8). Head suspension apparatus may be fixed to the top of the apparatus, for suspension of the patient if so desired.

Technique. The patient is given two stockinette vests to wear. The outer one sticks to the plaster and is used to bind the edges of the plaster, and the inside one is to enable the patient to change the vest. If necessary, Cestrofoam (a plastic sponge rubber bandage) is wound round the patient's trunk to protect against the sharp edges of the plaster and to protect the iliac crests, a possible bony area.

Two plaster slabs are prepared from 8-in. (20-cm) Gypsona bandages for reinforcing the back and front of the plaster. Five 8-in. (20-cm) plaster bandages should be sufficient, and should be quickly applied and well rubbed in. One bandage should be kept to apply once the outer vest has been cut 3 in. (7·5 cm) away from the top and bottom of the trimmed plaster. This bandage covers the turned over edges of the plaster. Sufficient plaster should be cut away from the lower edge to accommodate the thighs when the patient is in a sitting position. If the plaster is to extend to the sternal notch in front, an extra slab is required for the upper border, or an anterior pattern may be cut beforehand. The height of the front is the important factor in preventing flexion of the spine. The same

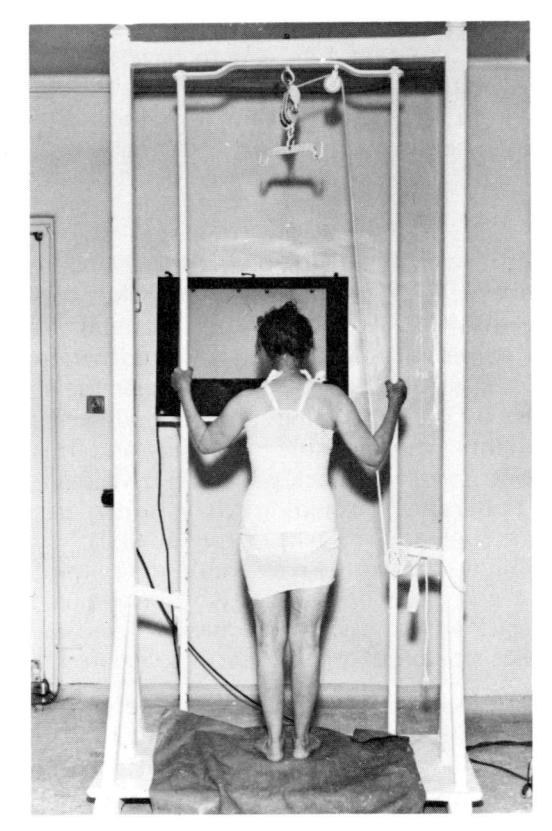

Fig. 8. Plaster jacket, showing patient standing on the Sayer's apparatus.

procedure can be carried out for a cast for a moulded leather, polythene or Goldthwaite jacket, but only one vest is required, and fewer and thinner slabs. The patient changes his vest by having the lower edge of another vest sewn to the upper border of the inner vest already on the patient. It is then drawn down under the plaster by pulling and easing the inner vest by the bottom edge.

Hip Spicas

These plasters immobilize one or both of the hips and include part of the trunk and the leg of the affected side, either to include the foot, or to end above the knee (Fig. 1).

Technique. The patient is supported under the shoulders, sacrum, knees and ankles on a hip stand or orthopaedic table such as the Hawley or Charnley apparatus, thus leaving the trunk and thighs free for plastering. The trunk is padded with sewn stretched felt, and the limb with plaster wool. The plaster patterns should be cut out first and reinforcing slabs prepared. The plastering starts around the pelvis and includes the hip. One joint is fixed at a time. When the hip has set, then the knee is fixed, and so on to the foot. The felt is turned over at the top edge of the plaster, and sufficient plaster is cut away from the pubic and rectal areas for nursing purposes.

Frog Plasters

With the advance and changes in surgery for the treatment of the congenital hip, frog plasters are not used so much these days. They extend from below the nipple line to the toes, bilaterally. The hips are held in abduction and external rotation. The hip stand is used for its application.

Batchelor Plasters

These bilateral leg plasters are also used for the treatment of the dislocated hips. The plasters extend from the tops of the thighs to above the malleolli and are joined together with one or two bars. These bars may be wooden or metal, and hold the hips in abduction and internal rotation. Care should be taken to see that the lowest ends of the plasters are well padded, preferably with felt strip. The advantage of this type of plaster is that the pelvis is free, so that it is much easier for the mother to keep the plasters clean. A hip stand is not necessary for the application, though it may be easier to maintain the position during application if it is used.

Leg Plasters

Below knee walking plasters are commonly applied in any Casualty or Orthopaedic Departments.

Technique. The leg is either covered with stockinette or plaster wool, special care being taken to see that the fibular head, ankles and heels are properly protected. The foot and ankle should, if possible, be in the neutral position to facilitate easy walking. A strong plaster slab is prepared posteriorly to extend from the toes to the upper part of the leg and incoporated with the 4- or 6-in. (10- or 15-cm) plaster bandages. Sufficient room is allowed to fully flex the knee; the toes being generally left free. It may be necessary to watch the circulation, especially after manipulation or surgery.

Long Leg Plasters

The same technique is used except that the plaster extends from the mid-thigh or even higher. An extra reinforcing slab is used to strengthen the knee. It depends on the purpose of the plaster as to whether the knee or ankle is immobilized first.

Walking Heels

There are a variety of walking heels in general use (see Fig. 9).

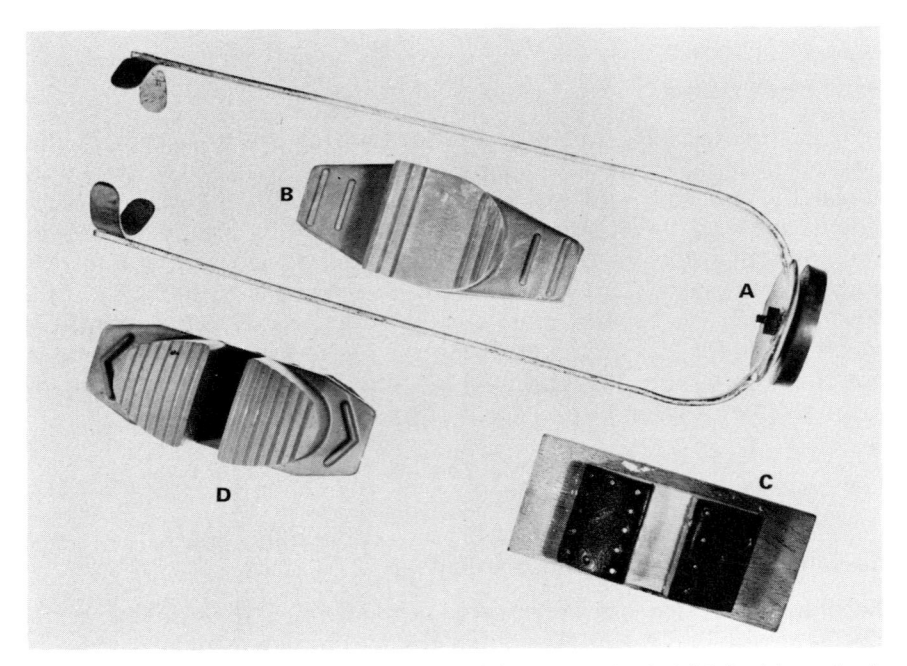

Fig. 9. Walking heels: (a) Böhler iron; (b) Zimmer heel; (c) left chinese heel; and (d) rocker heel.

Böhler iron. This heel is attached to bilateral metal shanks. The rubber heel is usually circular, but may also be rectangular. It is particularly useful when a plaster has to be applied with the foot plantar flexed, as it can be fixed long enough for the toes to clear the ground.

Wooden rocker heels. These are rubber covered rocker shaped heels, especially useful for the older patient who has difficulty in balancing.

Zimmer rubber heels. These probably wear the longest and are popular for children. They made in three sizes. Zimmers also make a type of rubber heel called a Chinese heel. This has a wider base and is made with a cleft in the middle for easy application.

Application of walking heels. The Böhler iron needs careful positioning; if the foot is at a right angle two fingerbreadths of space should be left between the top of the rubber and the bottom of the plaster. Two plaster bandages only are necessary, one encircling the leg covering the top bars of the iron (this should be firmly applied and well rubbed in) and the second one, applied round the iron, covering the front of the ankle and the point of the heel. Two loops of plaster are tucked in on either side between the iron and the plaster. If only one leg is in plaster, it may be necessary to put a temporary compensatory raise on the opposite shoe to equalize the length of the legs.

When applying any of the other walking heels two plaster bandages are always required; the first one is made into a thick pad and placed between the under surface of the walking plaster and the top of the heel (which is pressed into it), and the second plaster is applied over the front and back ends of the walking heel and round the front of the ankle. The plaster bandage needs to be well moulded when setting.

Plaster Boots

Some hospital departments keep a stock of plaster boots which are worn directly over a plaster. Although rather expensive they ensure a more natural gait and protect the plaster. Plaster boots can be made of either leather or canvas and should open down to the toe.

Minerva Jacket

The Minerva jacket is applied either for fractures of the cervical spine or after correction of a torticollis (Fig. 10). In either case the head and trunk are included, the face and ears being left free. Felt

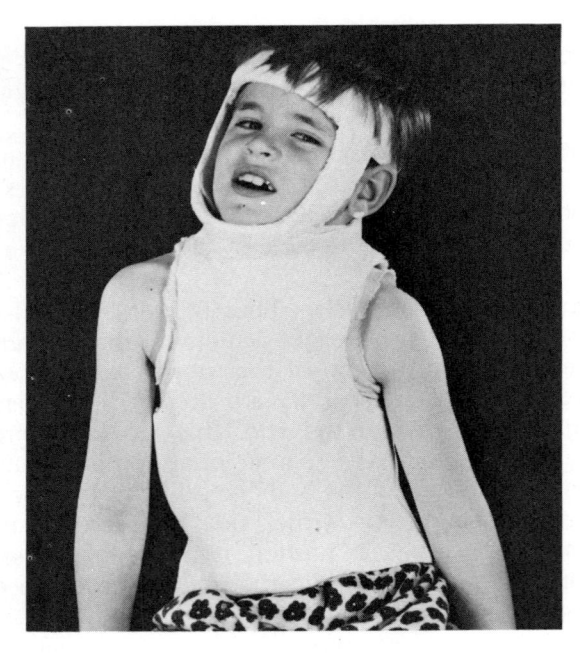

Fig. 10. Minerva jacket for a patient with right-sided torticollis. Note the rotation towards, and side flexion from, the affected side.

padding is used throughout and a selection of plaster slabs should be prepared. The position of the head after a tenotomy of the sterno-cleido-mastoid muscle should be rotation towards the affected side and side flexion away from the affected side. This position is manually maintained during application of the plaster.

Petrie Plasters

These plasters are sometimes known as 'broomstick' plasters and are used for patients with Perthe's disease (Fig. 11). An advantage is that the patient can stay at home, only coming into hospital at

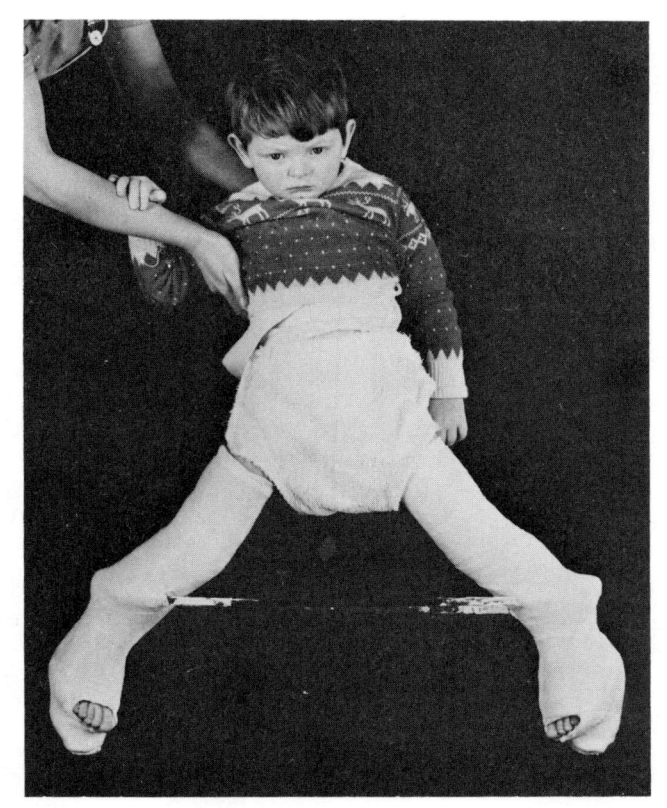

Fig. 11. Petrie plaster. Note the abduction and internal rotation of the hips, and the angle of the walking heels.

3-monthly intervals for a week's mobilization and reapplication of the plaster. The plasters are unwieldy and the patient needs the help of crutches.

Description. The plasters extend from the tops of the thighs to the toes on either side. They are joined by a broomstick cut to the correct length, or a pair of flat metal bars. The position of the limbs is of great importance. They should be maximally abducted, muscle spasm often being the limiting factor. The legs should also be internally rotated. The maintenance of both internal rotation and abduction ensures the correct position of the head of the femur within the acetabulum. The plastering needs to be strong and

17

carefully applied, with extra padding round the heel, ankles, knees and the upper edges of the plaster. Walking heels are applied when the leg plasters are dry. The application of the walking heels is not easy due to the rotation of the legs; Chinese Zimmer heels being most suitable although needing very thick plaster wedges placed under them, particularly on the outer sides of the heels. It is not uncommon for the plasters to be patched at intervals, especially when worn by very active children, and the plasters are under a great strain round the walking heels and at the junction of the bars.

Risser Jacket

When using this corrective form of splinting for a patient with a mobile scoliosis, it is necessary to understand the object of the exercise. Radiographs of the spine should be available, and the patient should have a clear explanation of the procedure. The Risser jacket is a combination of plaster, turnbuckles and hinges (Fig. 12).

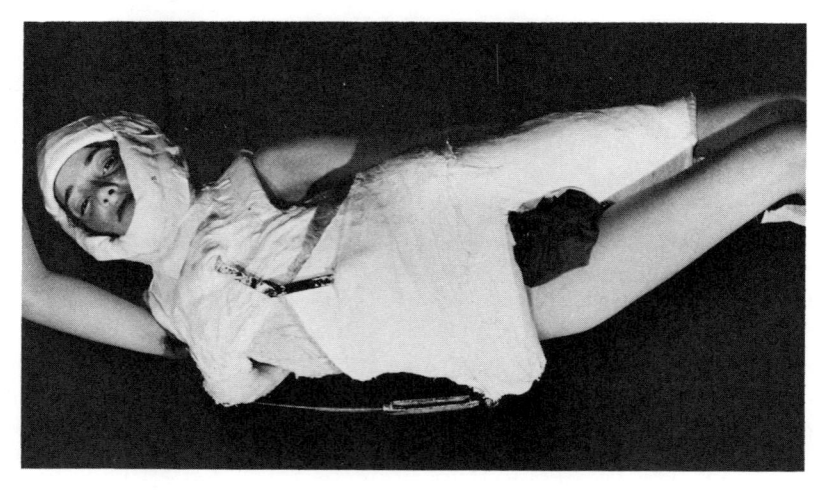

Fig. 12. A patient in a Risser jacket showing some correction, the turn buckle having been considerably unscrewed on the convex side.

It is applied in two stages with the patient supported on a framework table to allow as much freedom of the trunk, head and thighs as possible. The plaster extends from the chin and occiput to one knee, and one arm may be included as far as the elbow.

Technique. *First stage.* The patient lies on an adapted Goldthwaite-type table with facilities for applying traction and also support in the desired side flexion. The patient has a stockinette halter under the chin and occiput which is attached by its ends to a windlass at the top of the table. If the side flexion is too acute a manual pull may be necessary. Extensions are fixed to the patient's legs and tied to the bottom windlass. The patient is covered with stretched felt which is sewn carefully and firmly so that it is tailored exactly. The area of maximum pressure, over the greatest convexities of the curves should have two or three extra strips of felt attached, as should the iliac crests if prominent.

A number of strong plaster slabs of varying sizes should be prepared, five or six layers of plaster being sufficient for the head, trunk and hip. These are all incorporated in strong low plaster loss (L.P.L.) plaster bandages. The plaster should be well trimmed and the felt turned back over the edges when possible and the ears should be left free.

Position. In most cases the thoracic curve has to be corrected. The patient's lumbar compensating curve is exaggerated, the patient being swung to that side, and then the correction of the upper curve takes place by means of the turnbuckles and hinges.

Second stage. When the plaster is dry (usually about 5 to 6 days later) the next stage is carried out. At the level of the maximum correction of the upper or primary curve, the whole plaster is cut through surrounding the trunk. A large wedge should be cut out on the convex side. A turnbuckle is plastered in over the concave side and hinges are fixed centrally back and front, the area of opening where the wedge was removed closes up as the turnbuckle is unscrewed (this being done about two to three times a day). When the first screw is fully turned a second longer one is inserted, and a third one should be ready when the second is finished with. Progress is controlled by the correction achieved when measured by serial radiographs.

Third stage. When the desired correction has been obtained the plaster is filled in, the turnbuckes and hinges removed, a large window cut posteriorly: the patient now being ready for surgery.

Localizer Jacket

The localizer jacket is an extensive plaster which is applied on the patient with scoliosis prior to internal fixation, usually by Harrington's rods. Great care is taken to obtain the maximum traction from the occiput, chin and pelvis, at the same time producing lateral pressure on the apex of the greatest convexity of the curve to be corrected.

Apparatus. The apparatus used for the application of the plaster is the modified Goldthwaite traction table which gives adjustable support under the head, shoulders, pelvis, knees and ankles. A semi-circular metal rod is fixed under the patient in a line with the curve to be corrected. Through one of a series of holes in this localizer rod a bar is passed which ends in a round leather-covered pad, this is the point which is positioned at the area of maximum convexity of the curve. Sufficient pressure of this straight rod is applied to give the required correction.

Technique. The preparation of the patient, who should be adequately prepared beforehand, takes time and can be an ordeal. The following procedure should be followed:

(1) The patient should have a well-fitting cotton vest applied. Wide stockinette can be used and fastened over the shoulders with adhesive tape.

(2) The plaster extends from the chin and occiput to the greater trochanter level, so this area is covered with stretched felt sewn together. The felt pattern can be the same as that used for collars, but joined to the trunk portion.

(3) The patient's head is covered with a stockinette cap for protection.

(4) A stockinette halter with long side pieces is made and placed under the chin and occiput.

(5) The patient is lifted on to the table and positioned.

(6) A long canvas or nylon sling is placed lengthways under the patient, and is fixed to the windlass at the foot end of the table. The upper end has a loop and a transverse metal bar is passed through it. This bar is fixed to either side of the table just below the shoulders. The sling is tautinered from the lower end.

(7) Two 8-in. (20-cm) plaster bandages are applied to the patient's pelvis.

(8) A long 6-in. (15-cm) calico bandage is laid on either side of the patient reaching to about 6 in. (15 cm) above the waist. More

plaster is applied to the pelvis over the lengths of bandage, the part above the waist being turned over the plaster and incorporated in it. Very careful moulding must now be done over the iliac crest.

(9) When the plaster has set, the two lengths of calico bandage are tied to the foot end of the table, at the same time the head traction is fixed to the top end of the table. Both ends are tightened to the extent that the patient can just open his mouth.

(10) Plastering is now carried out, using a selection of plaster slabs to reinforce all areas, especially the junctions of the head and trunk plasters.

(11) When all the plaster has set the traction is released, the bar with the longitudinal sling is slipped out at the shoulder gap, and the sling pulled out from the bottom.

(12) The plaster is trimmed round the mouth and head, exposing the ears, under the arms, over the shoulders, and at the centre front and back, leaving these areas free for nursing purposes.

(13) The localizer pad is removed and the gap left is filled with plaster.

(14) The patient is returned to bed.

A traction belt can be used instead of side bandages. It is more comfortable for the patient if there is a thick felt pad over the localizer point. This plaster is usually re-applied with more correction after 2 to 3 weeks. The operation is carried out through a large posterior window.

Kites Plasters

Kites plasters are used in the treatment of the relapsed club foot. The foot reverts to the equino-varus position and needs to be reduced and held in the calcaneo-valgus position (Fig. 13). This can be done by first applying a below knee plaster to include the toes. The foot should be well padded and it is advisable to have an additional strip of felt encircling the heel and front of the ankle. This plaster should be allowed to dry completely before the next stage is carried out. A large wedge is marked on the plaster anteriorly and laterally and a horizontal line is marked across the midpoint of the heel. Using a handsaw, the wedge is removed and a cut is made across the marked line of the heel so that there is a complete division there. A small portion is left undivided on either side of the ankle. The anterior wedge is then gently closed, the foot being pushed up in the everted dorsiflexed position.

It will probably not be possible to completely close the wedge at first, in fact, it usually takes two manipulations to achieve this. When the maximum correction is obtained, that is, within the limit of pain, the divided plaster is reinforced. A single layer of plaster wool is wound round the heel and ankle, and then one small plaster bandage is applied over the wool. The inclusion of the plaster wool enables the plaster bandage to be easily removed for the second manipulation. The plaster can be left on for a few weeks after full correction is obtained, but more generally, a completely new plaster is applied with the foot in the over-corrected position.

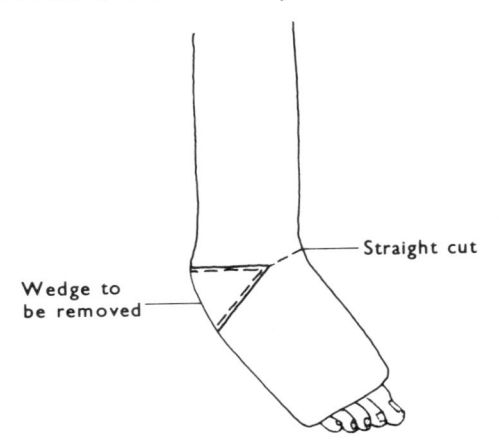

Fig. 13. Kite's plaster.

Plaster Night Splints or Removable Splints

There are several methods of making plaster night splints. Correct positioning and adequate padding of the limb is essential, as is also an understanding of the condition of the limb to be splinted.

Night splints for the leg. Ideally the patient should lie prone. The skin can be greased with Arachis oil. The leg should be measured and the plaster slabs cut accordingly, but always allow at least an extra 2 in. (5 cm), because the plaster muslin shrinks after immersion. Three plaster slabs are necessary for either a long leg or below knee splint. They should be applied quickly one after the other and well moulded. When the foot is included, two extra slabs are required, one extending on either side of the foot from the hallux, round the heel to the tip of the little toe. The other, on the inner side of the leg below the knee, round the heel to the fibular head. These two slabs ensure strength at the ankle, where there is most strain. If the plaster is well moulded, when it is removed from the leg after it has set, it should be smooth and shiny on the inside, and require the minimum of trimming. The splint may be made by the same method over stockinette instead of oil. The pattern of the leg may be cut from a wide roll of Gypsona and be applied in one piece. This is not usually so strong. The slabs in all cases should be five or six layers of plaster. If, however, plaster and Glassona bandages are used, only two to three layers of plaster slabs are needed with a covering of two layers of Glassona bandages (Fig. 14). This method makes a very strong light splint suitable for the rheumatoid patient.

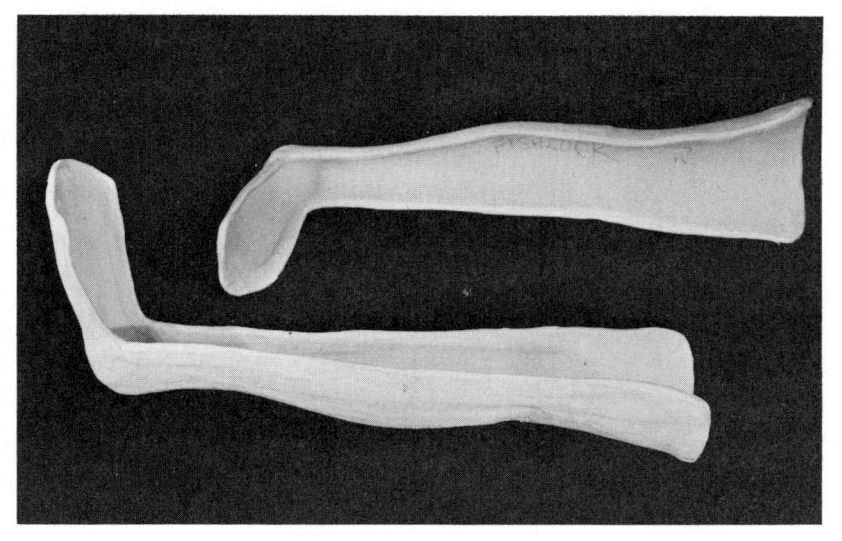

Fig. 14. Long leg plaster night splints, covered on the outside with one layer of Glassona.

Night splints for the hand. The carpal tunnel syndrome is often splinted at night (Fig. 15). These are simple splints to make and extend from half way down the forearm to either below the lower palmar crease or to the finger tips. In either case the patient rests the elbow on a table with the forearm supinated and the wrist extended. The area is measured, the plaster slab cut, and the forearm oiled. One

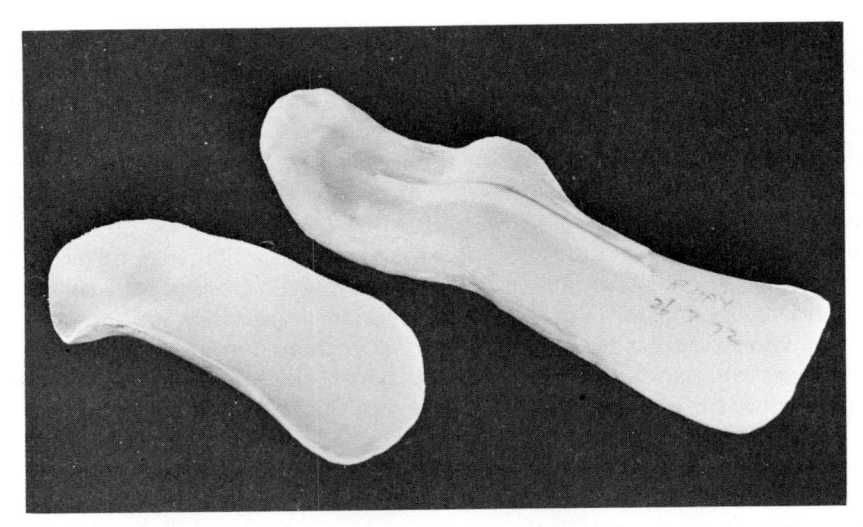

Fig. 15. Short and long plaster splints for night wear on patients with carpal tunnel syndrome. Note the tram-line reinforcement on the long cock up splint.

bandage is sufficient for the slab and any extra reinforcement that may be necessary. The slab is applied, removed when set and trimmed round the edges with a sharp knife. The patient should dry the splint in a warm place before wearing it.

Elbow splints. Elbow splints are made with a selection of slabs. The elbow joint should be at a right angle and the plaster is reinforced by a similar method to the ankle joint.

All night splints are best kept in position by crêpe bandages.

PLASTER CASTS

All moulded leather, polythene and Glassona splints are most satisfactorily measured by means of a plaster cast. Correct delineation and length of the limb or trunk can be obtained from the cast. It is also the most accurate way of showing bony points; this being particularly important for the instrument maker, as it enables him to build up the prominence on the filled cast. Over these prominences layers of grey felt can be attached to the plaster positive thus eliminating the chance of the leather or plastic material rubbing the skin.

Technique. The technique of taking a plaster cast is the same for limbs and the whole trunk.

Materials required. The following materials are required for plaster casts:

(1) An indelible pencil for marking any prominent bony point on the skin.
(2) Oil or petroleum jelly to cover the skin to be plastered, or, alternatively, stockinette stocking or vest.
(3) A length of wire to extend a few inches above and below the length to be plastered.
(4) Gypsona plaster bandages of the required width.
(5) A sharp cobblers knife.
(6) A bucket of warm water.

Procedure. The patient should be told about the procedure. The limb or trunk is usually covered with stockinette, any bony prominences first being marked with an indelible pencil. This mark is transferred to the inside of the cast, which, in turn transfers the mark to the filling. The length of wire is laid down on the outer side of the limb, or centre front of the trunk over the stockinette.

Correct positioning is extremely important. The optimum position of use must be employed whether the splint is for stabilization, weight relieving or protection. Plaster of Paris is then applied over the length of the limb or trunk and should be a few inches above and below the required length of the splint. This gives the instrument maker the necessary limits. Sufficient plaster is applied so that when it is removed the shape is maintained. The plaster should be of even thickness throughout.

A series of horizontal lines should be drawn with the indelible pencil over the length of wire which lies between the stockinette and plaster.

When the plaster has set, it is cut through, against the length of wire, with the cobblers knife. The wire is held in the left hand and it is gently pulled at the same time as the plaster is cut. The cast is then gently removed from the patient and then joined together by means of plaster bandages in such a way that the horizontal lines are in exact opposition with one another. One end of the cast is sealed off with a plaster of Paris bandage. The cast is finally labelled with the patient's name, and dated. It is now ready for filling.

A mixture of coarse pink plaster is made into a thick cream. The cast is held erect, a metal strut placed in the centre, and the plaster cream slowly poured in. Filling too quickly causes air bubbles to form. The outside plaster is stripped off once the filling has set, the name and date being transferred to it. It is found to be easier to strip down the same line used when cutting the plaster off the patient. The resulting filled cast, if to be used for a moulded leather splint, should be placed in a drying cupboard for 2 to 3 days at a temperature of 65·5°C. If the splint is a plastic one, it can be used for moulding straight away.

Casts of the neck for collars or of small joints, e.g. hand and fingers, or severe deformity such as kypho-lordosis, are best taken over oil. It is difficult to apply well-fitting stockinette over these areas. Some people also prefer to use oil when taking casts of the feet.

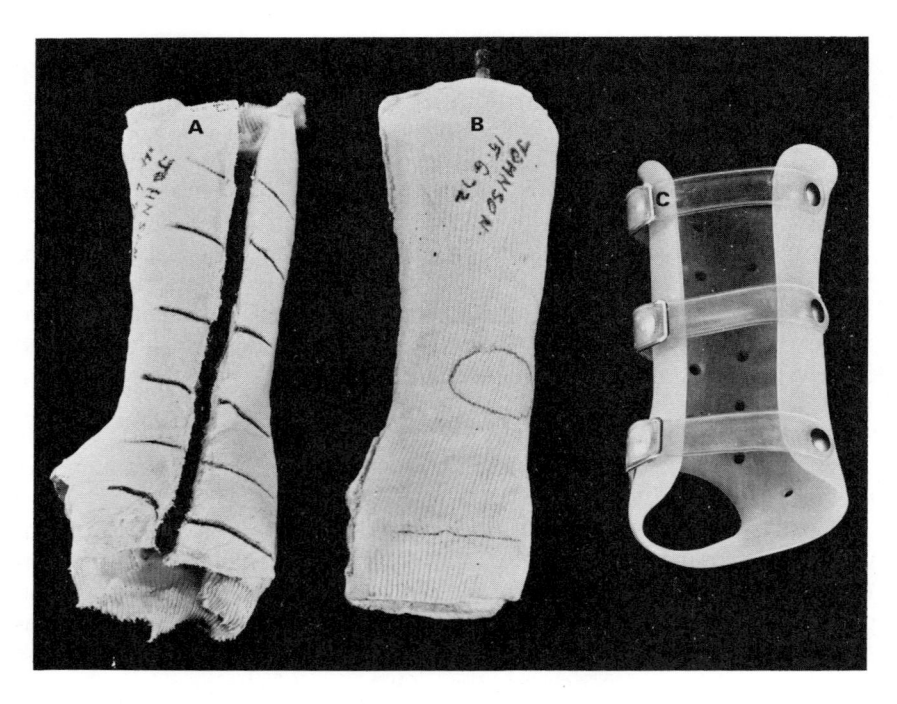

Fig. 16. Photograph showing: (a) the plaster negative after removal from the patient; (b) the positive; and (c) the finished polythene wrist support.

Lay On Casts

When one surface of the trunk needs to be cast it is not necessary to completely encircle the area, and plaster shells can be made. The Robert Jones brace (see p. 155) only needs a posterior lay on cast, that is, only the back is cast. The J. B. Mennell plates (see p. 173) incorporated in a corset or belt need anterior and posterior lay on casts.

PLASTER BEDS

This large piece of apparatus ideally needs a team of five operators: four to attend to the patient, and one responsible for mixing the plaster and, in fact, to be in charge of the operation. Considerable time is taken on the preparation of the bed, but the actual making of it should not take more than $\frac{1}{2}$ hr.

Preparation. Measurements of the patient should be carried out first, as follows:

(1) The length of the patient from shoulder level to gluteal fold.
(2) The length from the waist to external malleolus.
(3) The inside leg length, that is, from the groin to internal malleolus.

All these measurements should have the addition of an extra 4 in. (10 cm) to allow for shrinkage of the muslin. At the same time as measuring for the bed it is advisable to measure for the turning case:

(1) The length from shoulder level to external malleolus.
(2) The inside leg length from groin to internal malleolus plus 4 in. (10 cm) to each measurement.

Book muslin in pieces 36 in. long and 36 in. wide is used. The muslin is folded twenty-four times for each series of measurements. It will be noted that the bed is made in two halves, so that there is an overlap between the waist and gluteal fold. This ensures extra strength in a vulnerable area, when sufficient plaster has been cut away for nursing purposes. These two portions of twenty-four layers for the bed are divided into six portions of four layers each. The four layers are sewn together in each corner. The top and lower halves are arranged alternatively on a rack; they are so placed that the last one is the rectangular top one (which is the first one used). The lower half is split up the middle to the inside leg measurements.

Materials required
  (1) Twenty-four layers of sewn muslin cut to measurement.
  (2) One wide firm table for the patient, with a second one alongside.
  (3) A selection of sandbags.
  (4) A trolley laid with two large bowls capable of taking 20 pints (12 litres) (these should be on the top shelf).
  (5) The lower shelf should have one 2-pint (1·2-litre) measuring jug, three 7-lb. (3·15-kg) bags of superfine plaster of Paris, a tin of petroleum jelly gauze, a bottle of warm Arachis oil, an indelible pencil and some sharp cobblers knives.

Method. It is important that the patient knows something of the procedure beforehand, as the patient lies prone and is stripped, he cannot see what is being done.

(1) The patient should be positioned in the prone position, with the spine straight, and the forehead resting on a sandbag, so that the face is not actually resting on the table. A sandbag under the front of each ankle, to allow a little flexion of the knees, and a soft pillow or flat sandbag under the abdomen if there is a lordosis present. The arms can hang over the side, resting on a stool, with a roll of wool under the arm to prevent discomfort from the edge of the table.

(2) The patient should have the whole trunk and legs oiled, and petroleum jelly gauze placed over the hairy areas. There should be a protective covering put over the head.

(3) Whilst the patient is being prepared, the plaster can be mixed. Ten pints (6 litres) of warm water is measured into one bowl. Plaster is poured into the water [approximately 1 lb. to 1 pint (1 kg to 1·3 litres)] until a fairly thick and smooth cream is obtained.

(4) When the mixture is ready, it should be twice the original amount in the bowl. The muslin patterns which should be on a rail adjoining the trolley, are passed, in turn, through the plaster cream, and handed over to the operators, two on either side of the patient. They place the patterns on the patient, smoothing gently but firmly from the centre outwards to exclude air bubbles. This procedure continues until all forty-eight layers of muslin are passed through the cream. It may be necessary to make a second bowl of plaster cream.

(5) The plaster should be setting on the patient; when it can be

knocked, the area to be cut away is marked with an indelible pencil. This is necessary all round the edge, and the central area from the coccyx to the leg cleft.

(6) The bed is labelled with the patient's name and is then carefully lifted off the patient and laid on the adjoining table (Fig. 17). Whilst the patient is being washed, the bed is trimmed with the knives. A flat edge is cut before the plaster gets too hard, even so it is sometimes difficult to do so at the coccygeal area as it is very thick. When the cutting is complete the bed is tried on the patient to make sure that sufficient plaster has been cut away.

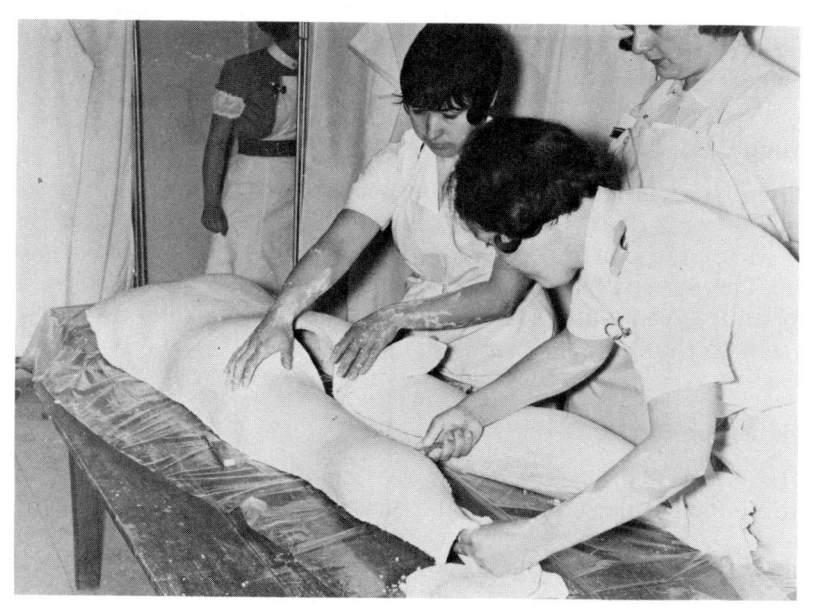

Fig. 17. Plaster bed at the trimming stage.

(7) The bed is turned over and should be smooth and shiny inside. If there are any wrinkles or uneven areas, they should be rubbed away, and then the whole area should be polished with pieces of wet Gypsona plaster bandages. This is an excellent way of using up odd pieces of Gypsona patterns or bandages. The edges of the bed should be smooth, although occasionally it is necessary to bind the edges.

(8) The bed is then dried in a heated cupboard (65·5°C) for 2 days.

(9) Nursing is made easier if the bed is mounted on wooden blocks.

Note: extension bows can be fixed, by means of plaster bandages, to the legs of the plaster bed, so that foot pieces can be attached to the extension bows. Alternatively the legs of the plaster bed can be made to extend to the toes. It is, however, difficult to make the plaster feet comfortable. The whole bed can be lined with Gamgee wool or white lint. This is more hygienic than having no lining. It is possible to make a plaster bed with a series of plaster slabs especially if only one or two operators are available. These beds tend to be heavy and not so finished. Plastazote sheets, $\frac{1}{4}$ in. (6 mm) thick, can be used as the first layer of a plaster bed, they make smooth linings and give resilience.

Turning Case

When the patient has become accustomed to the plaster bed, usually after 2 days, the turning case is made. The procedure is the same as for the plaster bed (p. 27), except that the pattern is in one piece. The patient has been through the operation once, and as he is lying supine, can watch all that is going on. The turning case is dried and sent to the ward.

Murk Jensen Plaster Bed

The Murk Jensen or lateral plaster bed (Fig. 18) is used for treating ideopathic scoliosis in the baby. It is only used at night.

Method. The baby lies on the side of the concavity of the main curve with a sandbag supporting the trunk at either end of the curve. This helps to open up the curve during the plaster application. When the bed is made the baby lies on its opposite side, or side of the convexity of the curve, so that in effect the curve opens up with the fulcrum at the maximum convexity. There is no reason why the position in the construction of the bed should not be reversed, except that the baby does not always tolerate a sandbag at the maximum convexity of the curve, as it literally would hang over it.

The baby's skin is oiled, and a series of plaster slabs applied. They extend from the shoulder to mid thigh. It is easier for the mother if the bed is mounted on a shallow wooden frame, so that pillows for

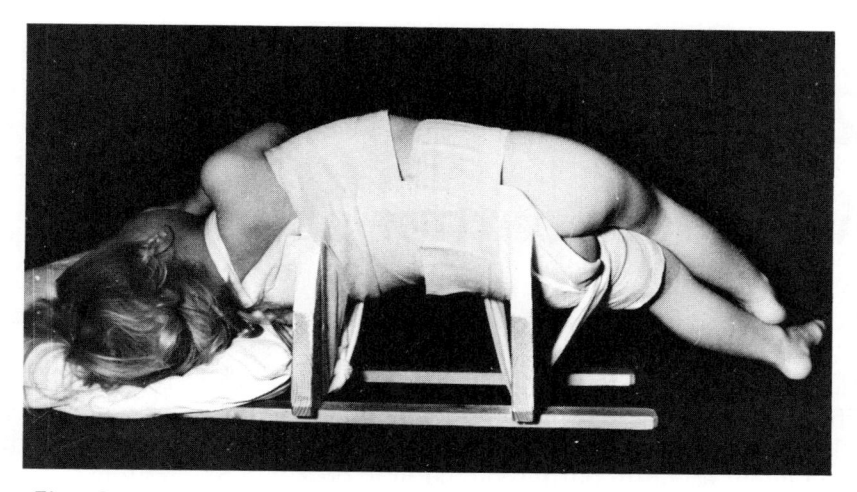

Fig. 18. Murk Jensen plaster bed, showing the patient lying on his side with the convexity of the bed approximating with the concavity of the curve.

the head and legs can be used. A canvas sling with an armhole can be used as an alternative.

PLASTER FOR AMPUTATION STUMPS

Amputation stumps are now generally covered immediately after operation by plaster of Paris caps. This ensures comfort for the patient, a reduction of phantom pain, and the firm, even pressure and immobilization ensures quick healing and a good shape for the stump. A temporary walking appliance can be attached to the plaster before the fitting of the eventual prosthesis.

Application. Two strips of Elastoplast may be fixed to the stump, one dorso-laterally, and the other anterio-laterally; these help to keep the plaster stable. Elastic Gypsona bandages are applied to keep an even pull, only one or two are required as they are coarser than the normal bandage and take considerably longer to soak.

2
Moulded leather splints

Moulded leather splints may be used to rest any part of the body. The making of these splints is a long process and always involves the taking of a plaster cast. The taking of a cast is necessary to obtain a completely accurate outline of the limb or trunk. Some splints, such as the walking caliper, are a combination of moulded leather and metal.

An understanding of the correct position of the limb is necessary before beginning on the cast. It must be remembered that the position chosen should be both one of rest for the affected joint, and one which allows maximum use of the adjacent joints. Any bony abnormality should be noted and marked with an indelible pencil on the skin. This mark is transferred to the inside of the plaster cast, and so on to the outside of the filling. The filled cast, when stripped, is dried in a heated cupboard at 65·5°C for about a week before being transferred to the workshops for the leather work to be commenced. It is necessary for the positive to be completely dry, as the leather has to be nailed on to the cast.

The leather should be soaked in warm water for 1 to $1\frac{1}{2}$ hr until it is pliable. It is then stretched and moulded over the cast and nailed in position for 1 to $1\frac{1}{2}$ days. When the leather is dry, it is removed and is ready for rough fitting on to the patient (Fig. 19). At this stage the leather can be trimmed if required, and even re-moulded. It is then returned to the workshops for finishing. This involves lining with chamois leather or glace calf, polishing with beeswax polish, and reinforcing with duralumin.

Moulded leather splints are comfortable and durable. They are absorptive, can be re-lined and repaired. They are firm without being too hard, and do not have hard edges, but they do take longer to make than plastic ones.

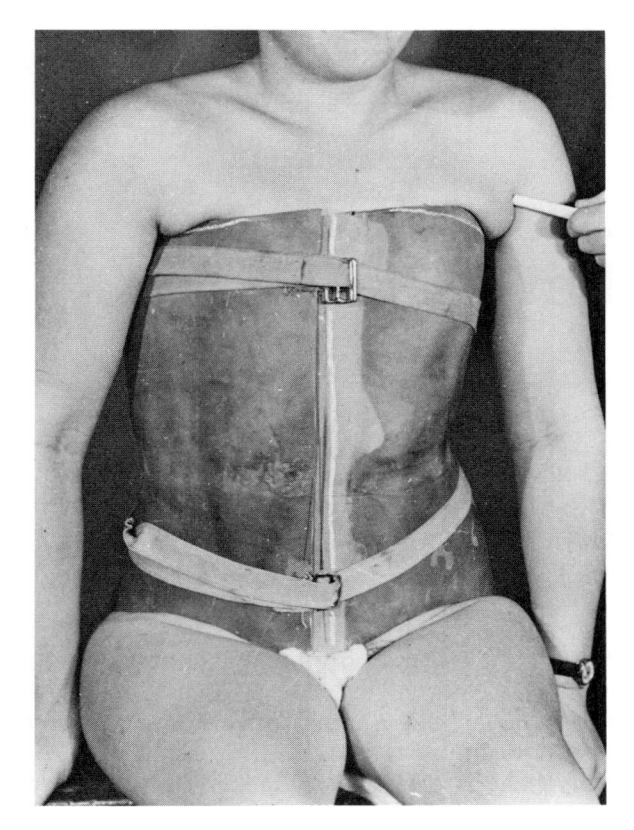

Fig. 19. Moulded leather jacket being fitted in the rough. Note the chalk lines for showing trimming required and junction of the overlap.

3
Splints made from synthetic materials

Polythene has become a very popular material for splints for almost every part of the body (Figs 21 and 22). It is a solid polymer of the gas ethylene and is suitable for semi-rigid splints. It is made in varying thicknesses of $\frac{1}{8}$, $\frac{3}{16}$ and $\frac{1}{4}$ in. (3, 4·5 and 6 mm). Sheets of 2 ft × 7 ft are suitable for use.

The required amount is cut from the sheet of polythene and placed in an oven until the temperature reaches 180° F, usually 4 min is sufficient. In that time the polythene should become transparent. It is then moulded on to the cast, where it is left for 15 to 30 min, when it can be removed, cut where necessary, and the edges polished.

It is particularly important that the cast should be inspected before the polythene is applied, so that any prominent bony points can be built up with felt pads.

Polythene splints are cheaper than leather, quicker to make, and are easily cleaned—but like all plastic materials they are non-absorbent, so that hot, greasy skin may not take kindly to it. They can be lined with foam rubber if necessary. Velcro straps are usually used, or in the case of collars, adjustable plastic clips.

All polythene splints need a plaster cast. Polythene collars (Fig. 20) are particularly popular, as are bed splints for rheumatoid knees, and also for the haemophiliac patient with knee involvement.

The Anti-Pressure Heel Splint

The polythene splint (Fig. 23) is lined with thick adhesive foam and extends from below the knee to the toes. The heel portion is exaggerated in size and the heel is slung. The support is given above

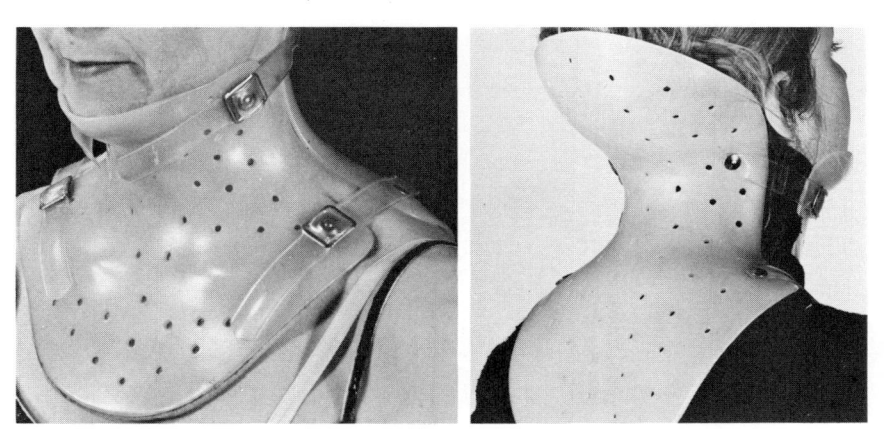

Fig. 20. Polythene collar.

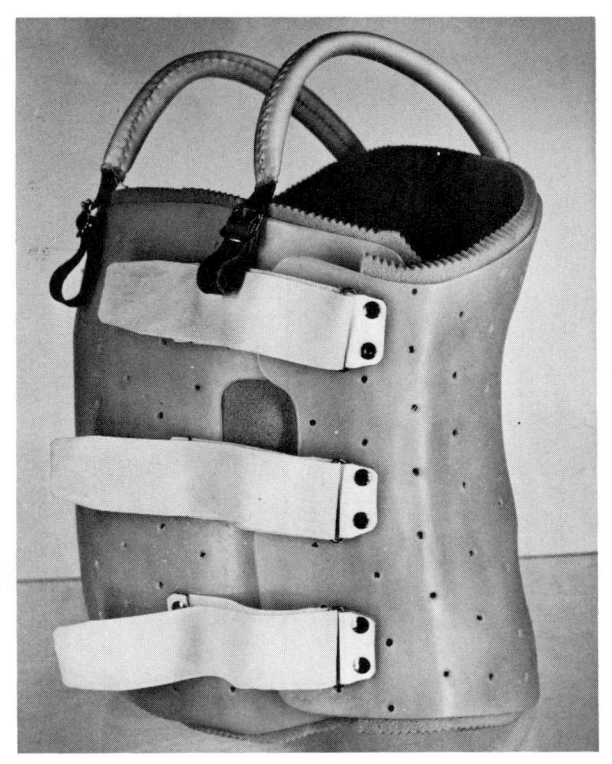

Fig. 21. Polythene jacket with shoulder straps.

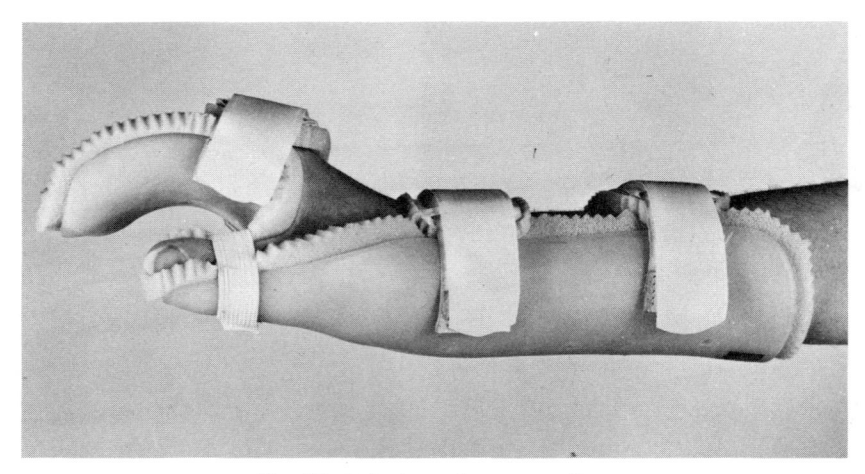

Fig. 22. Polythene forearm splint.

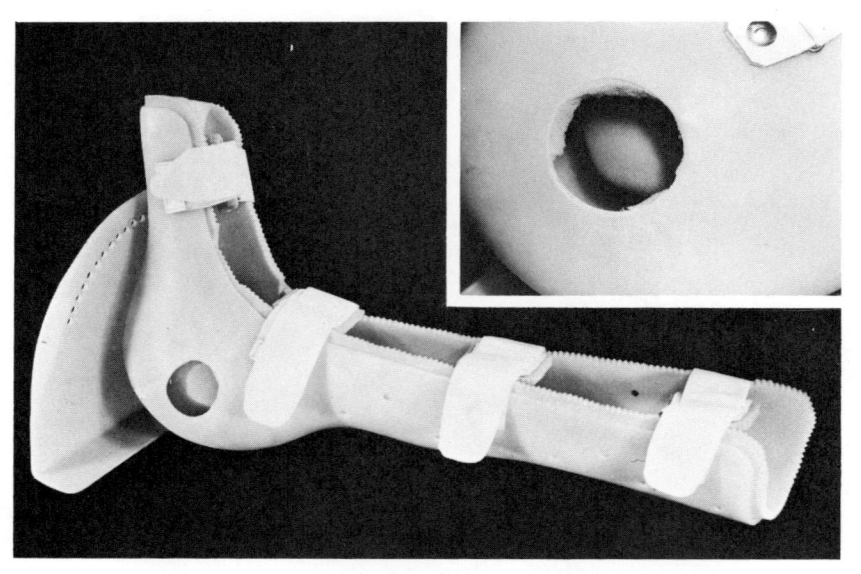

Fig. 23. Anti-pressure splint. Note that the heel is slung with no contact surrounding it.

the ankle and the sole of the foot. A round opening is made on either side to avoid any pressure on the malleoli. The foot piece is attached to a perforated semi-circular polythene plate with a ledge on the straight border. This allows the amount of rotation required to be fixed and maintained. Velcro straps are used to keep the splint in position.

These splints can be kept in stock in one or two sizes. A cast for the original is made, but padding will have to be applied to the heel and ankle before casting is carried out.

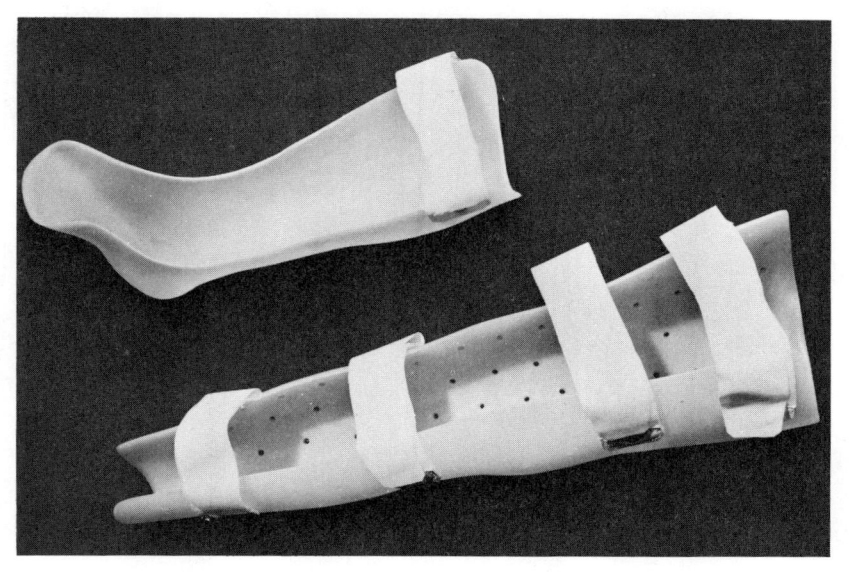

Fig. 24. Night splints for the foot (top) and knee (bottom).

Leg Splints

Concealed polythene splint for the flail leg. This is a splint worn next to the skin, under the stocking and inside the shoe, and is made as inconspicuous as possible (Fig. 25). A plaster cast is required of the whole leg and foot with the level of the knee joint marked. The thigh is completely covered with polythene which extends anteriorly to just below the knee and posteriorly above the knee. This allows for flexion with stability. It is lined with foam rubber or leather and has a soft edge at the posterior top. The back of the thigh is strengthened with polypropylene, at either side of which the shanks are attached. There are ring locks for flexion. These can be covered with chamois leather to protect the stockings. The posterior calf and foot to just below the metatarsal heads are enclosed in a polythene shell, also lined. If the patient's calf is thinner than the opposite side, a plastazote false calf can be made to enclose the back half. Thus a flail leg is stabilized, flexion of the knee is possible, and a raise on the shoe does not affect the length of the splint.

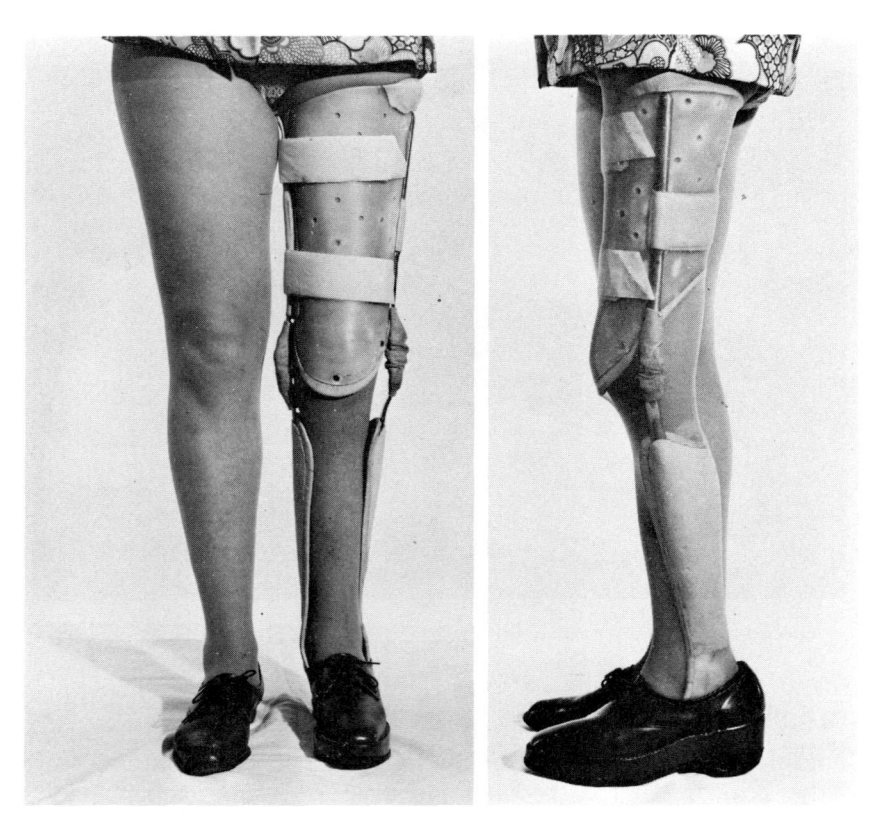

Fig. 25. Concealed polythene splint for flail leg. Front and side view.

GLASSONA

This useful plastic splinting material is a combination of cellulose acetate and acetone. The bandage is made of a mixture of glass and cellulose acetate fibres knitted into a silky coarse stockinette to form a bandage. This in turn is immersed in acetone, which should be in a tin with a hinged lid, not an open bowl, as it is imflammable in this state. The bandage should be immersed in acetone for 2 s to a depth of not less than 4 in. It should not be squeezed but the excess acetone should be allowed to drip into the tin.

The bandage should be applied with sufficient tension to allow easy moulding, and preferably immediately after application of the last plaster bandage. The heat from the plaster during crystallization will speed-up evaporation of the solvent, and so hasten setting time. It takes 20 min to harden, and is completely hard when it is odourless. A warm hairdryer accelerates the drying. It is non-inflammable when hard, water resistant, exceedingly strong, light in weight, and translucent to X-rays.

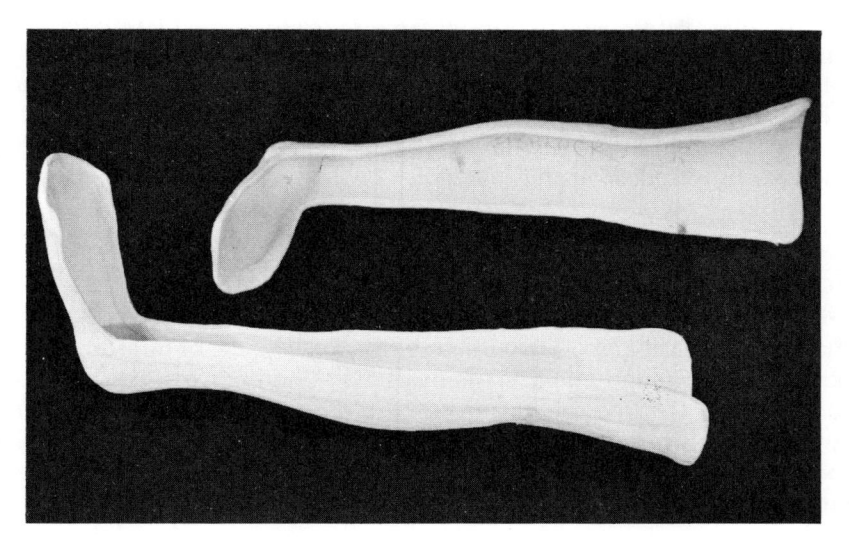

Fig. 26. Plaster day and night splints covered with Glassona.

Uses. If Glassona is required for a splint, it is best to take a cast and make the splint accordingly. It is often used to reinforce plaster night splints (Fig. 26), when it is only necessary to make a very light plaster shell covered with one or two layers of Glassona.

It can also be used at the top of small childrens' plasters, so that the area covered with Glassona can be washed.

PLASTAZOTE SPLINTING MATERIAL

Plastazote splinting has become very popular as it can easily be handled in a hospital department. It is very light in weight and can be scrubbed and even put into a washing machine. It is easily cut with a knife and so can be reduced in size if necessary.

Plastozote collars are especially satisfactory, but occasionally there is a skin reaction, and some patients find the material too hot.

Plastazote consists of foamed polyethylene of closed cell construction. It is non-toxic and of low flammability and is resistant to common acids. It is resilient and supports in a cushioned manner. It is available in 24 × 36 in. sheets; thicknesses varying from $\frac{1}{4}$ to 1 in. (6 to 25 mm).

Equipment. A hot air circulating oven is necessary. The temperature should reach 140° C before use.

Adhesives such as 'Bostick' or 'Evostick' are useful, as also are Velcro fastenings of different sizes.

A sharp knife is essential, and for a very smooth finish to the edges, a powered scouring machine (20 in. high speed hand scourer) is useful.

A punch or stapler may also be used to fix fastenings.

Technique. While the oven is heating to 140° C the Plastazote can be prepared. The bottom of the oven should first be covered either with the easy release paper provided with the sheets of Plastazote, or dusted with French chalk. This prevents adherence of the Plastazote to the oven. Outline the pattern required on the Plastazote sheet and cut with a knife or pair of scissors. The Plastazote expands 1 in. per foot on heating therefore there is no need to oversize the pattern outlined. Place the pattern in the oven for not less than 5 min, longer periods will cause no harm providing the temperature of the oven does not exceed 150° C.

If desired, cover the limb with stockinette, but the pattern can be applied directly on to the skin. It is wise to check that the surface heat is not too hot before application. As soon as the Plastazote is brought into contact with the skin, gently stretch and mould it. Plastazote starts to set after about 20 s.

Remove the splint after 3 to 4 min and trim the edges with either a sharp knife, an emery wheel or No. 1 glass paper. The splints are best kept in position by prefabricated Velcro straps.

Plastazote Splints in General Use

Cervical collar. The $\frac{1}{2}$-in. sheeting is used and the pattern shown in Fig. 27 is satisfactory. One Velcro fastening is needed.

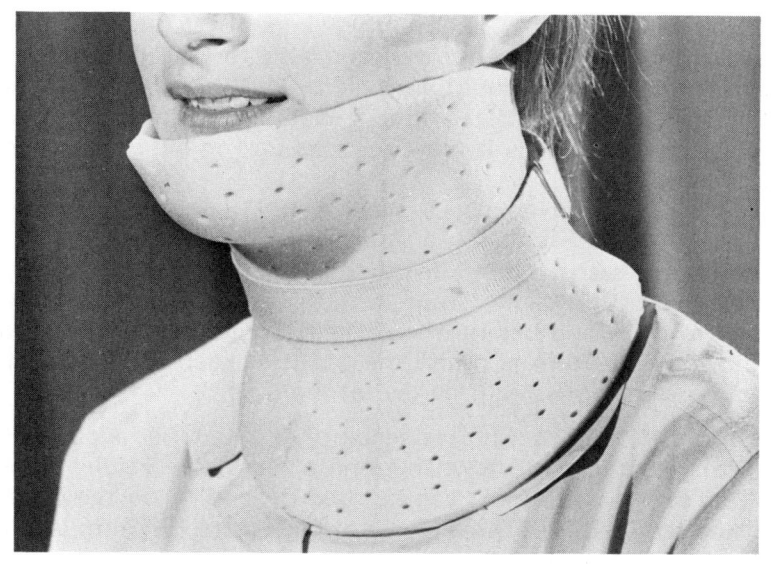

Fig. 27. Plastazote cervical collar.

Forearm and wrist supports. The $\frac{1}{2}$-in. sheeting is used with two Velcro fastenings (see Fig. 28).

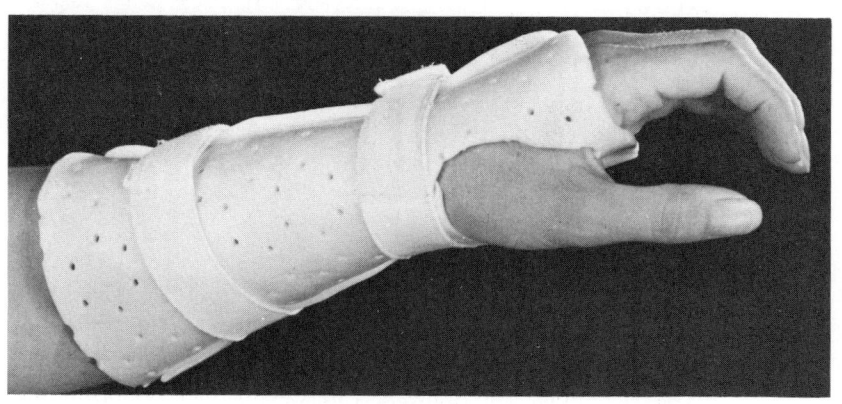

Fig. 28. Plastazote wrist support.

Jackets. These supports can be reinforced with strips of solid polyethylene sheeting $\frac{1}{16}$ in. (1·5 mm) thick. When a reinforced jacket is required, two layers of $\frac{1}{4}$-in. (6-mm) Plastazote sheeting is required and the polythylene strips placed 3 to 4 in. (7·5 to 10 cm) apart between the two $\frac{1}{4}$-in. (6-mm) layers of Plastazote. Allow an extra minute or two in the oven and also for the moulding. One important precaution should be taken. The polyethylene retains a greater heat than the Plastazote and should *never* protrude beyond the Plastazote, otherwise it may cause a burn on either the operator or patient.

Jackets may be melaminated, when $\frac{3}{4}$-in. (18-mm) sheeting will be used.

Speed is necessary in moulding such a large splint to the body. The setting time is the same, so it is necessary to have an operator standing in front and behind the patient. Some people find it easier to wind a crêpe bandage round the trunk to keep the Plastazote in contact with the patient during the setting time.

Shoe insoles (Fig. 29). The resilience of the material is particularly comforting to the patient when using a Plastazote insole. Sheeting 1 in. (2·5 cm) or less thick, can be used depending on the depth of the insole required. Cut three pieces of Plastazote 12 × 4 in. and heat two of these pieces. Place the unheated portion on the floor in front of the seated patient. When one heated portion is ready, place it on

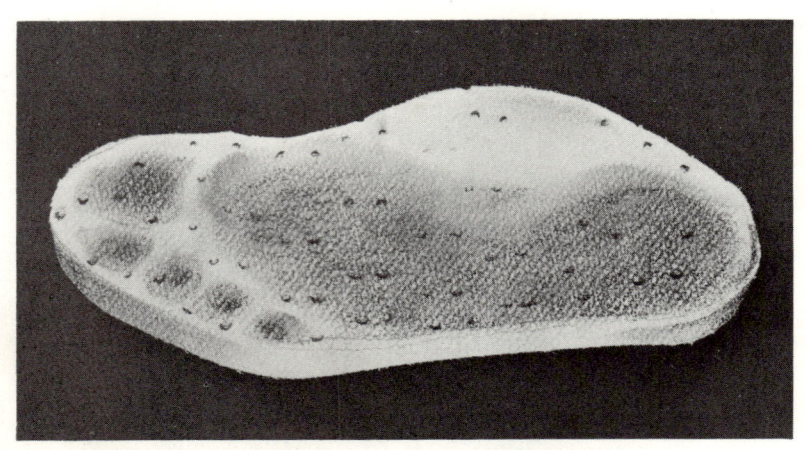

Fig. 29. Plastazote insole. This shows a $\frac{3}{4}$-in. (2-cm) thick plastazote insole suitable for use in a surgical shoe. Note the total weight transference of the foot.

top of the unheated portion, dust the top with French chalk, and stand the patient with full weight on one foot if possible, for 2 to 3 min. During this time the foot should be held, the sides being pressed upwards and the arches moulded.

Repeat the process for the other foot. When cooling has occurred it will be necessary to trim and pare the insole to fit the shoe. These insoles need to be replaced after 6 months of continuous wear.

Light splints for the leg and arm can also be made.

Plastazote Casting

Plastazote can be used instead of plaster casts for spinal jacket measurements. Plastazote sheeting of $\frac{3}{8}$ or $\frac{1}{2}$ in. (9 or 12 mm) thick is used and moulded rapidly round the patient. When cool it is removed and joined together by plaster bandage, and then the Plastazote shell is filled with plaster in the usual way.

PRENYL

This is a semi-rigid, pink plastic material of pleasant appearance. It is particularly suitable for small splints such as cock-up splints, opponens splints, heel caps and arch supports. It is strong and unbreakable, and is non-allergic and non-toxic. Most patients like the softness next to the skin and its resilience. It does not need any lining, and it is washable.

Technique for hand splint. Prenyl is available in sheets of 14 x 27 x $\frac{1}{8}$ in. or 14 x 27 x 1 in.

(1) Measurement is obtained by drawing an outline of the hand on the sheeting allowing an extra $\frac{1}{2}$ to $\frac{3}{4}$ in. (12 to 18 mm) extra all round.
(2) The marked material is dipped in water (at 60°C), and then cut with a pair of scissors.
(3) The splint is then moulded on to the forearm and hand and held in position for a few minutes. Any pieces can then be trimmed if necessary.
(4) The splint is held in position for 20 min by means of an elastic bandage.

(5) Any fastening tabs that have been allowed for in the pattern can be heated in the hot water or placed under a hair dryer and pulled to the required length. Alternatively Velcro fastenings may be applied with Prenyl cement.

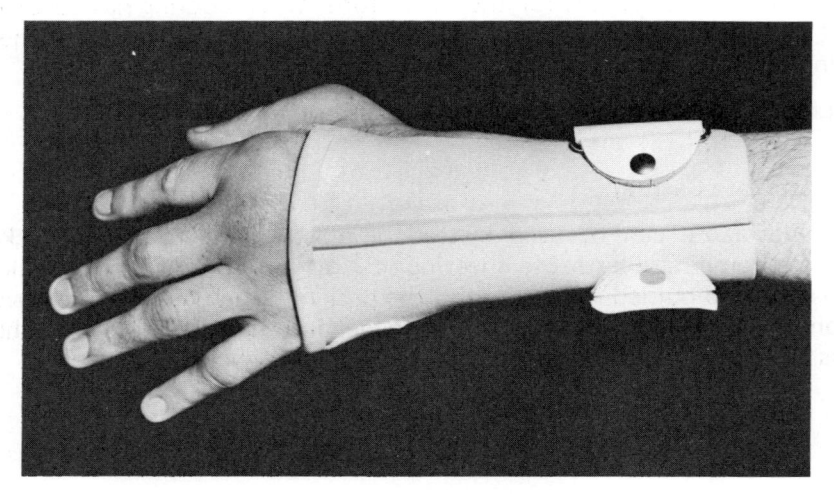

Fig. 30. Prenyl wrist support.

This splint can be remoulded at any time. It can be perforated with a leather punch, and is easily riveted to aluminium or steel.

FORMASPLINT

Formasplint, also known as Darvic splinting, is white in appearance, rigid, strong, washable, lightweight and inexpensive. It is available in sheets of $36 \times 24 \times \frac{3}{32}$ in. It is composed of unplasticized vinyl (PVC). It is extremely rigid and special attention should be paid to the temperature when a splint is being constructed. This thermoplastic material needs to have the edges smoothed. The smoothed surface can be scratched by sharp projections, or damaged by acids.

Technique. The material should have the traced outline of the required splint made directly on to it. It is then heated in water at a temperature of 90·5°C. If hotter than 90·5°C the gloss finish deteriorates, and if the heat is less it becomes brittle.

The material is cut with a conventional coping saw or fret saw, preferably with five fret teeth. Holes can be drilled with an ordinary twist drill. The material is moulded directly on to the patient, and maintains the imposed shape on cooling. It can be lined with polystyrene, Copydex being used to make it adhere to the splint. In the first instance a sharp knife can be used to cut the edges, the blade being held at right angles to the material. Coarse sandpaper can also be used to smooth the edges, followed by a finer sandpaper for a smoother finish. The resulting splint is extremely rigid, but has extreme pliability during moulding. It is not successful for hand splints.

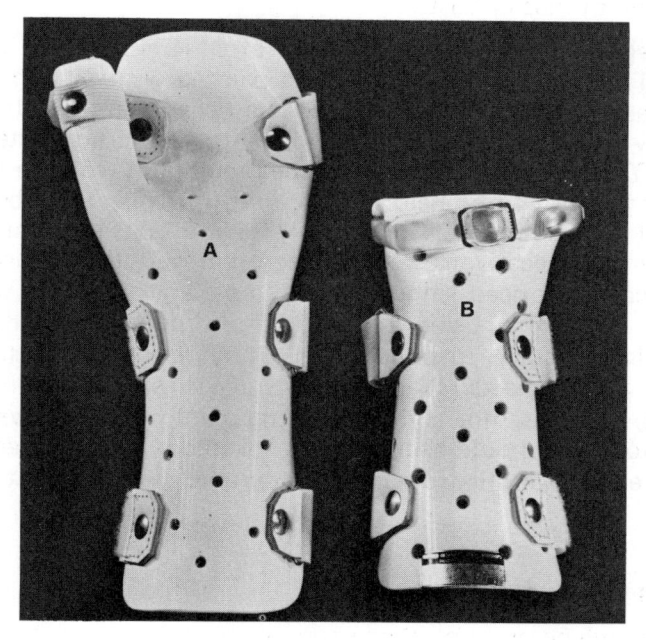

Fig. 31. Formasplints: (a) resting splint; and (b) splint for daily use.

POLYPROPYLENE AND POLYTHENE APPLIANCES

The above material is rigid and thermoplastic with a good chemical resistance and has electrically insulating properties. These materials have a high melting point. Boiling water will not soften or alter their shape after being moulded. Plastic materials are the easiest of all for use in the manufacture of appliances. They are mainly used for the type of splinting required for immobilization of the joints or the correction of limbs. It is light in weight when shaped to the plaster cast and concave and convex shaping adds to its inflexibility and strength. It can be purchased in pink and white coloured sheets varying from $\frac{1}{8}$ to $\frac{1}{4}$ in. in thickness.

On this type of splinting, the cast and subsequent mould is of great importance. The appliance will be no better than the cast on which it is moulded.

Preparation of Plaster Casts

The negative cast should be sealed after it is removed from the patient. The inside of the cast is then painted with oil or grease and liquid plaster of Paris is poured into the negative mould. It is often extremely helpful if a metal rod is put into the liquid plaster before it is set. This not only strengthens the mould, but will give a bearing point for the cast to be held in a vice or, in the case of a body cast, the metal protruding at each end will form an axis for the moulding spit. When the negative casing has been removed, the surfaces of the positive cast will need smoothing. It is easier to do this while the plaster is still damp, using a sharp knife, a spoke shave or Surform tool. It is necessary to build up all bony protruberances, such as maleoli, fibula heads, iliac crests, clavicles, prominent spinal processes, epiglotis, ulna styloids and the point of the elbows.

The moulding should then be well covered with stockinette. This is to prevent the plastic from cooling too quickly on contact with the plaster.

Moulding of Splints

Polypropylene and polythene can be shaped by two methods: (a) vacuum moulding, and (b) laying on a cast by hand. The technique for the latter is that it should be laid flat on a base of French chalk in an oven heated by gas or electricity (although infrared ray has been found to be more successful). When the material has been heated, and takes on a translucent appearance, strips of stockinette or any other material that will stretch in breadth and length should be put on each end of the plastic material in order that the operative may, with gloves, mould the heated substance. The plastic can then be lifted out of the oven and moulded on the prepared cast. The edges should be tacked in order to prevent shrinkage with cooling.

Some General Rules

It is important that great care should be taken in trimming the edges of the appliance when cool. The outer aspects of the moulding should be well smoothed and rounded. The plastic should be cut away at joints which require to move freely. A spinal supporting appliance should be cut well away at groins and under the axillas to enable comfortable sitting and movements of the arms. Appliances for the cervical spine should be cut to avoid pressure on the ears and shaped above the occipital protruberance. It is a mistake to make the chin cup too deep. The crevasse section of the collar should be wide enough to prevent movement. The width over the shoulders should allow for the arms to move above the head.

Casts for hand splints should be taken in the position of strength, and in cases of appliances for fractured scaphoids and those to restrict movements of the thumb, casts should be taken with the thumb in opposition.

Working type wrist and hand splints should be trimmed along the palmar crease and well behind the metacarpel heads of the dorsal aspect, in order that the hand may be clenched.

As the material is not porous, it will need a generous amount of ventilation holes.

Methods of fastening include plastic straps with adjustable press fastenings, buckles, which are the most convenient as these dry easily when washed. Velcro is an excellent method for fastening large appliances, such as leg or spinal supports. It is sometimes safer to fasten a hip spica and any applicance in which immobilization is vital, with leather straps and single pronged harness buckles fastened securely to the appliance with copper rivets. Fastening bilateral hand splints needs a great deal of thought. The strap endings need rather large loops whether made in Velcro or plastic strapping in order that very deformed fingers can grip them and the patients apply and remove the splints themselves.

4
Hand and finger splints

SMALL FINGER AND THUMB SPLINTS

Mallet Finger Splints

Mallet finger splints (Fig. 32) are usually of four types:

(1) Maleable metal.
(2) Polythene.
(3) Perspex.
(4) Frog splints.

These are used for a ruptured long extensor tendon, or mallet finger (sometimes called a cricket splint). The terminal interphalangeal joint is held in hyper-extension, and the interphalangeal joint in slight flexion. It is usually worn for 6 weeks, and should not be removed during that time. A selection of sizes are usually kept in stock.

Polythene finger splint (Fig. 33). This is an alternative splint which holds the terminal interphalangeal joint in hyper-extension. It may not be so easy to keep on and strapping may be added for that reason.

Perspex finger splints. Strips of Perspex, varying from 2 to 4 in. (5 to 10 cm) long and $\frac{1}{2}$ in. (12 mm) wide can be kept in stock, together with the spirit lamp for heating. The Perspex can then be held over a flame for a few minutes until it is warm and soft, and then moulded to the required shape. It is usually held in position on the palmar side of the finger by strips of $\frac{1}{2}$-in. (12-mm) strapping.

Frog splint (Fig. 34). This splint is made of malleable metal lined with sponge rubber, which clips round the finger at both extremities,

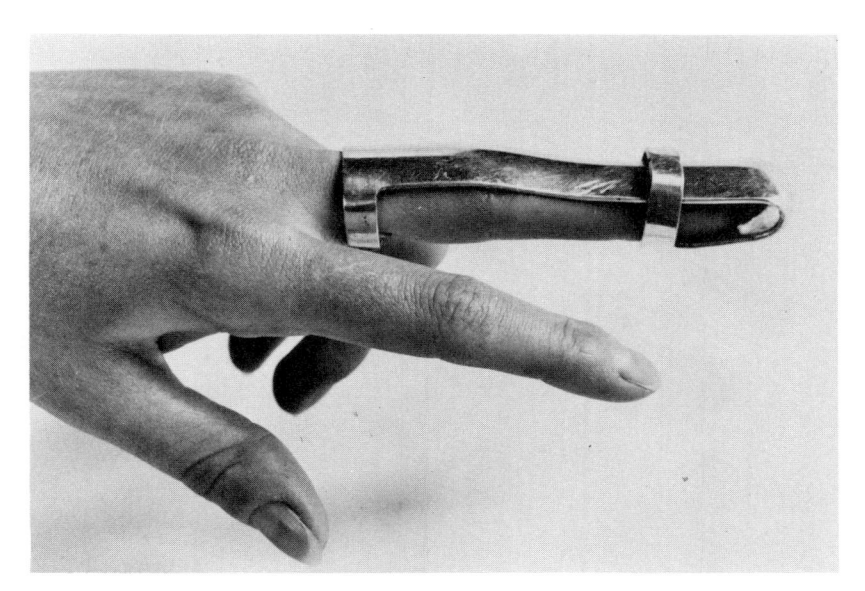

Fig. 32. Mallet finger splint.

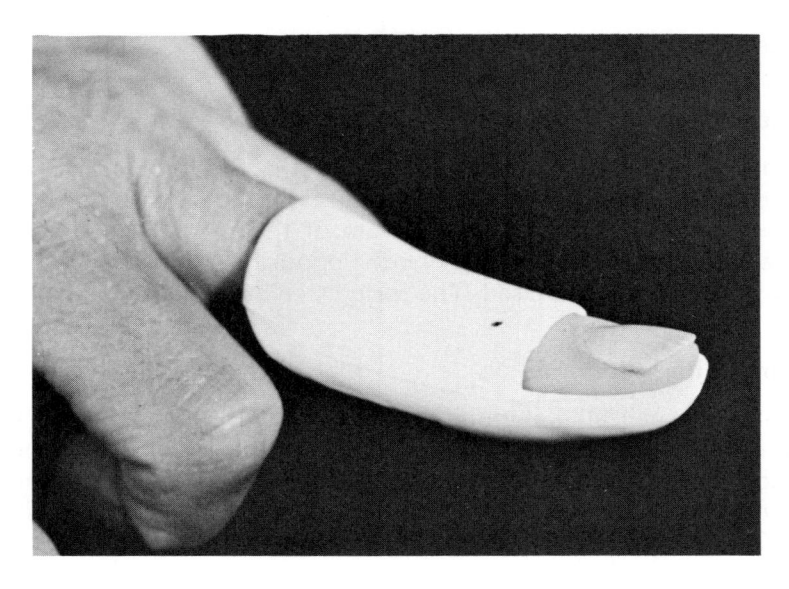

Fig. 33. Polythene finger splint.

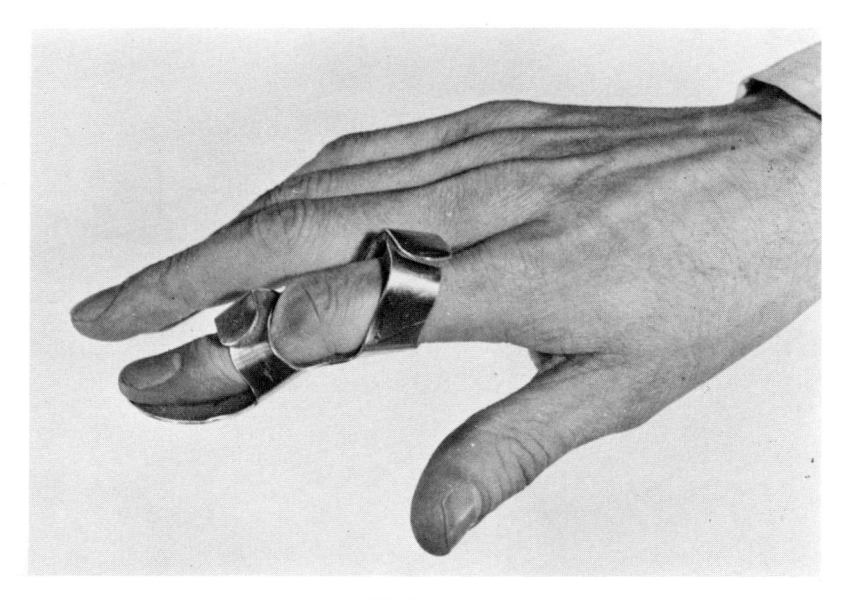

Fig. 34. Frog splint.

again hyper-extension of the distal interphalangeal joint is advised. These splints are made in a selection of sizes.

Armchair Splint

This is a delicate type of lively splint (Fig. 35), and is designed to give extension of the first interphalangeal joints. All lively splints are made with a wire coil at the fulcrum of the joint. This allows free flexion and extension, thus giving the opposing group of muscles the opportunity to be exercised. The spring steel is 22 gauge.

Zimmer Finger Splinting

Strips of malleable aluminium approximately $\frac{5}{8}$ in. (15 mm) wide and 18 in. (45 cm) long, and covered on one side with adhesive sponge. These splints are used a great deal in Casualty departments. The malleable aluminium strips can be cut with a pair of scissors, and moulded to the required shape. They can incorporate all the joints of one finger and the wrist, and are fixed by strips of 1-in. (2·5-cm) strapping (Fig. 36).

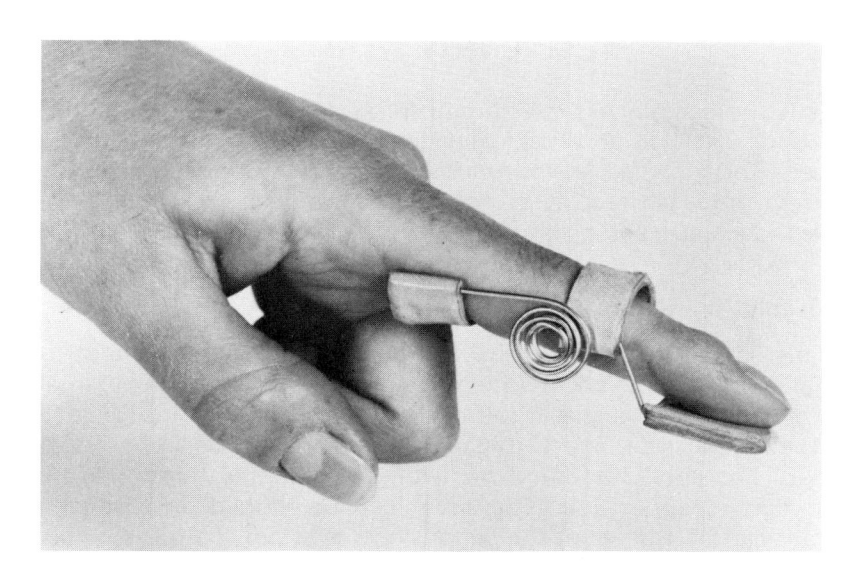

Fig. 35. Armchair splint.

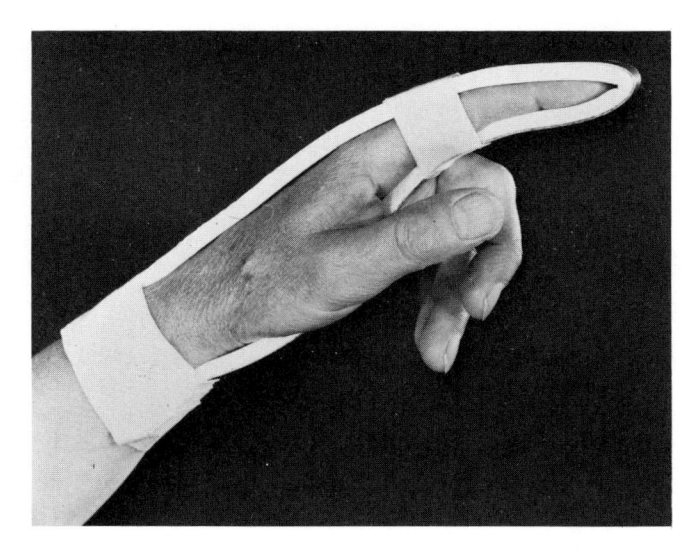

Fig. 36. Zimmer finger splinting.

OPPONENS SPLINTS

This is the name given to a thumb splint designed to hold the thumb in opposition and abduction, i.e. the thumb lies opposite the index finger. This position is the one of use, as the index finger can be brought into contact with the thumb, and so used for grasping objects such as a pen or knife.

Malleable Aluminium

This small, light and easily applied splint is made of a strip of metal $\frac{3}{8}$ in. (9 mm) wide, which encircles the hand just proximal to the metacarpal–phalangeal joints (Fig. 37). It has a 2-in. (5-cm) gap on the palmar side, and is joined to an encircling band of metal by a bridge. The encircling band of metal encloses the thumb and holds that digit in opposition. The splint can be slipped on through the palmar gap. A tracing of the hand is necessary for the measurements.

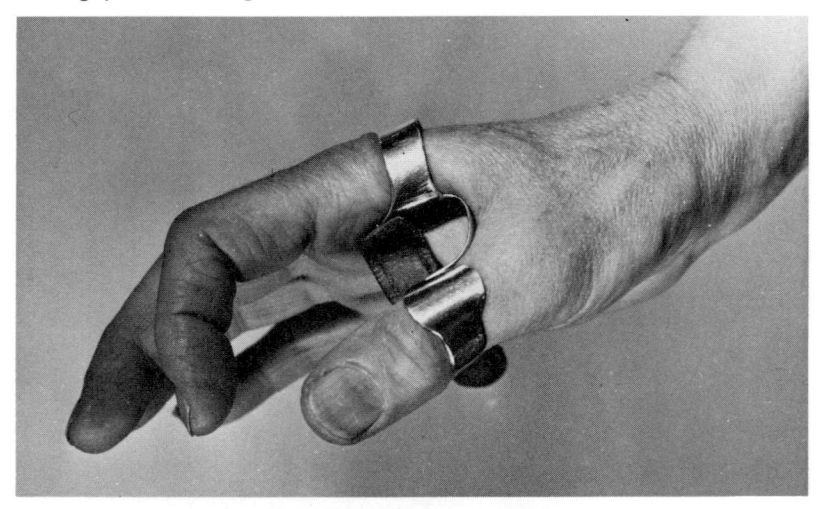

Fig. 37. Metal opponens splint.

Leather Opponens Splint

A leather (lined) circular band encloses the thumb, and is joined by a narrow leather strap to a wider lined leather band round the wrist (Fig. 38). It *must* be seen that the strap joining the thumb and wrist is kept on the palmar side of the hand. This is a comfortable splint, but unless the intervening strap is kept in position, it is useless. The leather can be lined with thin sorbo rubber, and a tracing of the hand is used for measurements.

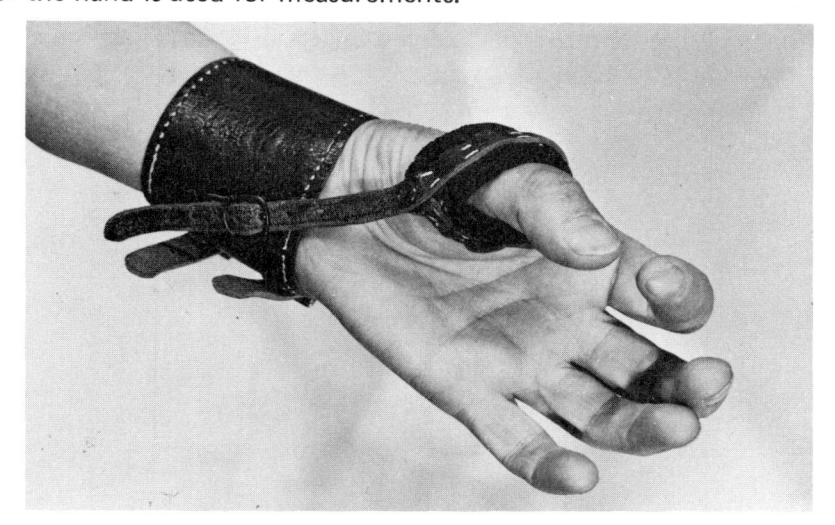

Fig. 38. Leather opponens splint.

Polythene Opponens Splint

A splint can be made of this plastic material which maintains the thumb in the opposed position. A plaster cast has to be taken first.

Moulded Leather Opponens Splint

This is an alternative material to the polythene, and is suitable for patients who do not tolerate plastic materials. Plaster casts are necessary, but this type of splint takes longer to make and is usually fitted 'in the rough', that is before it is lined, polished and reinforced.

The Glove Opponens Splint

A metal bridge between the thumb and first finger can be attached to a glove, thus maintaining the desired position.

Spider Splint

This name is given to a five finger splint for correcting digital extension. The five spring steels which are joined at the base of the thumb, lie across the back of the hand and end in metal bands which half encircle the palmar aspect of the fingers (Fig. 39). This is a neat and easy splint to apply and wear. A tracing of the hand is required.

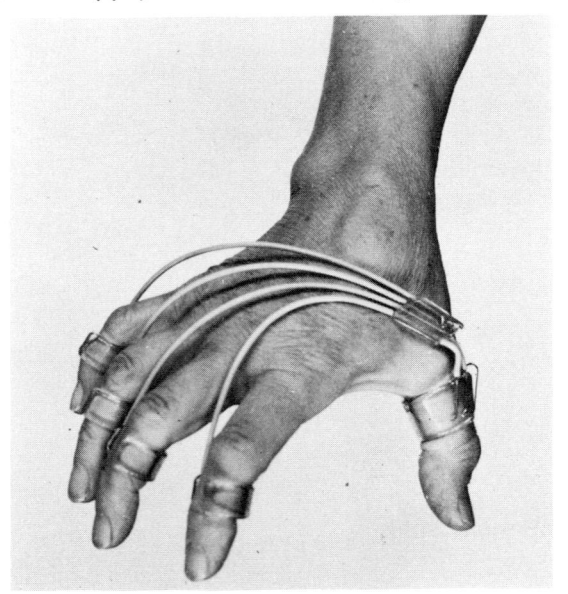

Fig. 39. Spider splint.

LIVELY SPLINTS FOR THE HAND

Ulnar Nerve Splint or Knuckle Duster

A knowledge and understanding of the deformity is essential here. The deformity due to an ulnar nerve palsy consists of hyperextension of the metacarpal phalangeal joints and flexion of the interphalangeal joints of the fourth and fifth fingers. Hence the splint is designed to give flexion of the metacarpal phalageal joints and extension of the interphalangeal joints (Fig. 40). A rigid splint may be worn with a small round metal palmar bar, leather covered, joined at each end. Two bars lie on either side of the knuckles, thus maintaining flexion of these joints and encouraging extension of the interphalangeal joints. More usually the double bars are joined at each end by means of a wire coil, which allows movement of the interphalangeal joints. The palmar bar is hinged and can be opened to allow application of the splint. When necessary an extension on the radial side can be added to maintain opposition of the thumb.

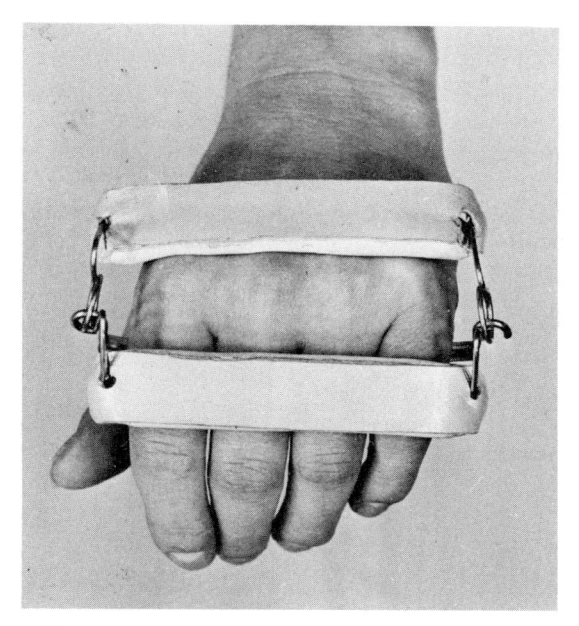

Fig. 40. Ulne nerve splint, or 'Knuckle duster'.

Median Nerve Splint

The deformity due to median nerve palsy is one of the 'flat hand'—the great disadvantage being the inability to oppose the thumb. Any of the opponens splints can be worn (see Figs 37 and 38).

Radial Palsy

The deformity consists of loss of extension of the wrist and metacarpal phalangeal joints, thus allowing use of the strong flexors of the hand and fingers. There are many different types of radial splints of the lively variety. The principle is the same, that of resting the wrist and fingers in extension, while allowing active flexion of the opposing joints.

Bryan Thomas Lively Splint

The Bryan Thomas lively splint is designed to give extension to the wrist and fingers, at the same time as allowing flexion to both wrist and fingers (Fig. 41). It may also have a thumb extension to help with the opposition. These movements are controlled by three coils of wire which are incorporated in the main framework. There is a padded metal bar, approximately 2 x 4 in. (5 x 10 cm) wide, which lies on the dorsal aspect of the hand, and an elliptical band of wire

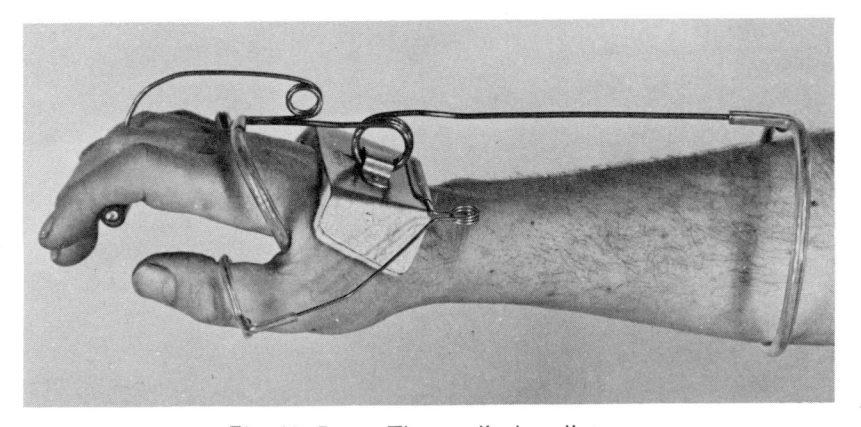

Fig. 41. Bryan Thomas lively splint.

encircling the metacarpal joints. These two stable parts are joined by the wire which has a coil with four turns on the dorsal band, and extends to a smaller coil of two turns in the middle of the encircling band of wire on the dorsal aspect. The smaller coil is extended to a cross bar which lies in front of the fingers, the wire pressing between the middle and ring fingers. The thumb extension goes from the radial side of the lower border of the dorsal bar, and has a small coil of three turns, and ends in a circular band which encircles the thumb. The wire for the main structure is 16-gauge spring steel, and that of the thumb a smaller gauge. The large circular wire enclosing the forearm, and that encircling the interphalangeal joints are covered by plastic tubing.

The Bryan Thomas lively splint is very light, easy to apply, durable, and easy to work. The measurements are best taken by a tracing of the hand, together with measurements of the circumference of the forearm in front of the elbow, the circumference of the hand at the level of the interphalangeal joints, and the circumference of the thumb at the terminal metaphalangeal joint.

Camp Steeper Radial Splint

This lively splint is made of steel spring wire covered in thermo-plastic tubing. It has a nylon palmar bar and wrist trough (Fig. 42). It may have finger extensions fitted to the palmar bar by means of wire coils.

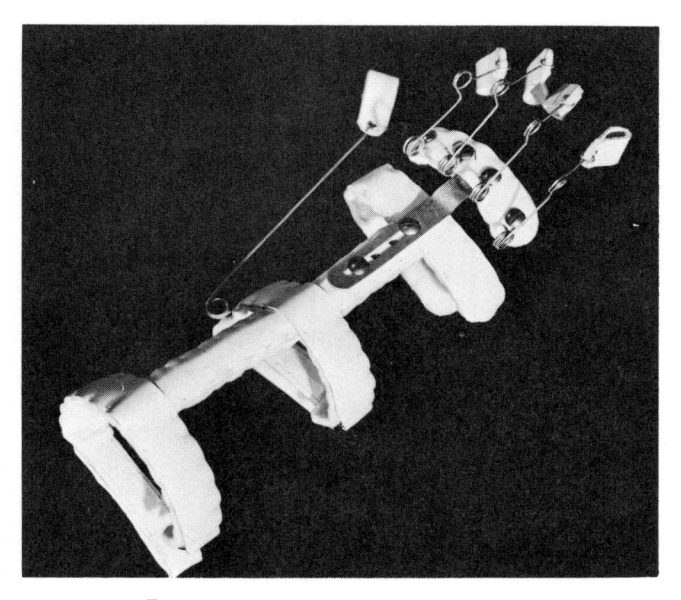

Fig. 42. Camp Steeper radial splint.

Leather Radial Splint

This splint incorporates the metal cock up splint with leather finger cap extensions. The whole splint is made of leather and elastic or rubber pulls for the fingers (Fig. 43). It is somewhat clumsy, but is durable and comfortable.

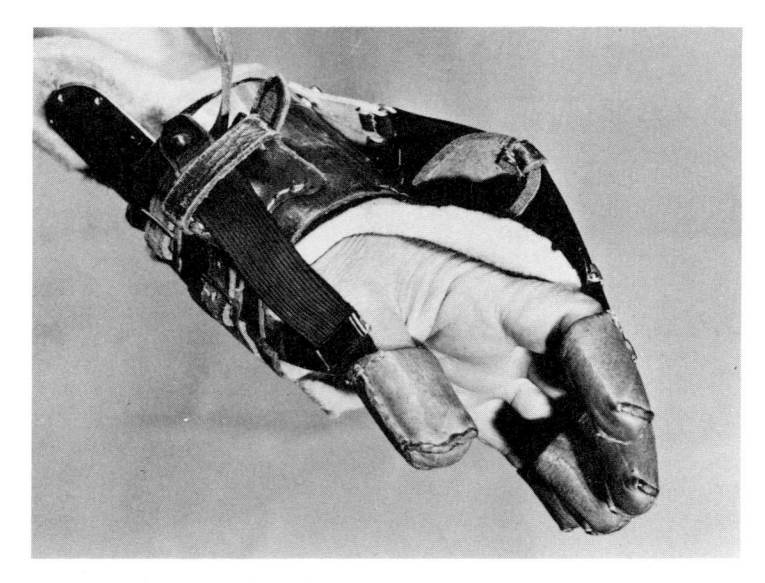

Fig. 43. Leather radial splint.

RHEUMATOID BRACES FOR THE HAND

The use of functional static and functional dynamic braces for the rheumatoid hand has been advocated. These braces can be constructed on the spot, and should not take longer than $\frac{1}{2}$ hr provided the basic materials are at hand.

Brace construction. The components are cut from a sheet of 16-gauge duralumin (Fig. 44). Adhesive felt and Velcro fastenings should be at hand. The braces must be strong enough to stabilize joints and allow full function of active joints. They should also be light-weight and, above all, comfortable. They are often used complimentary to surgery. The principle of the functional static brace is to stabilize some joints, and encourage movement in the other joints.

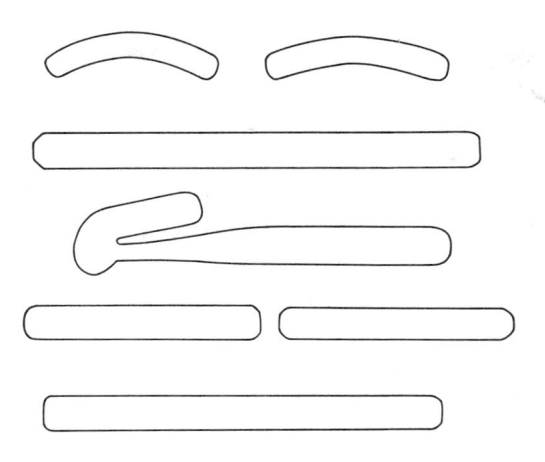

Fig. 44. Basic metal components.

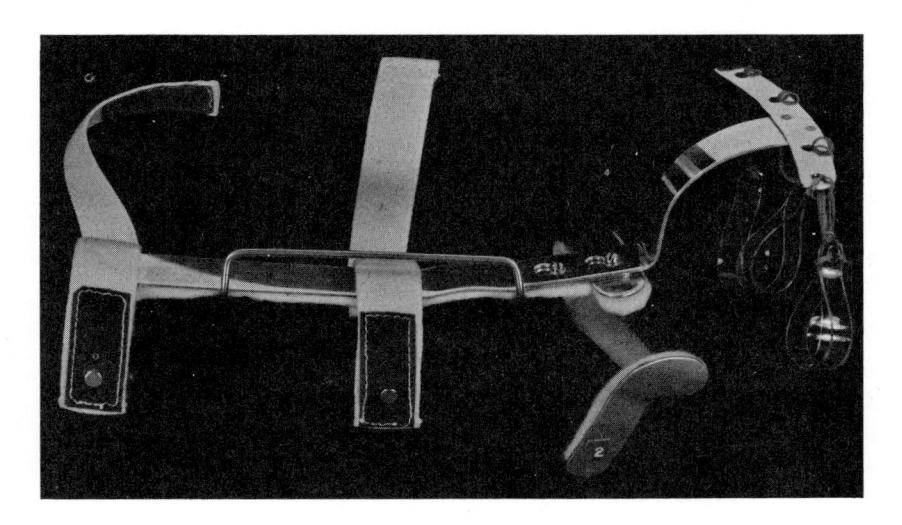

Fig. 45. Standard long opponens brace with metacarpal phalangeal extensor assist.

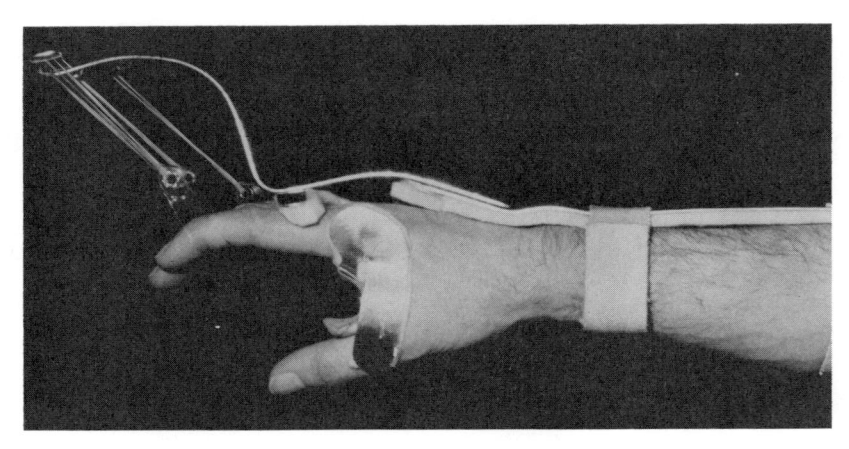

Fig. 46. Correction of proximal interphalangeal joint contractures using standard long opponens brace with metacarpal phalangeal control and proximal interphalangeal extensor assist.

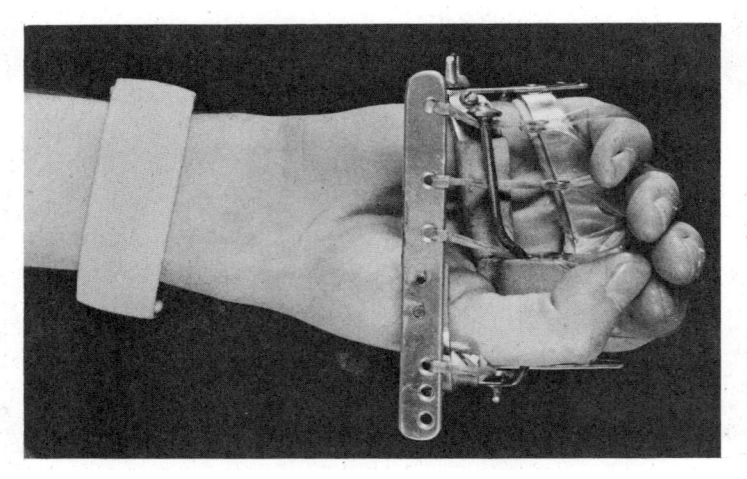

Fig. 47. Proximal interphalangeal flexor assist brace. Note the reverse lumbrical bar and the roller bar across the palm controlling the direction of the pull of the elastic assist.

Figure 46 shows the use of a standard long opponens brace preventing extension at the metacarpal phalangeal joints, and exerting continuous elastic pressure at the proximal interphalangeal joints.

Figure 47 shows the long opponens brace with proximal interphalangeal flexor for assistance. This also shows the offset extension bar to prevent, or control the ulnar deviation of the fingers.

Figure 48 is another view of the same splint, but shows the reverse lumbrical bar, and the roller bar across the palm, controlling the pull of the elastic assist.

The long opponens brace with a C-bar maintains the thumb in opposition to the index finger.

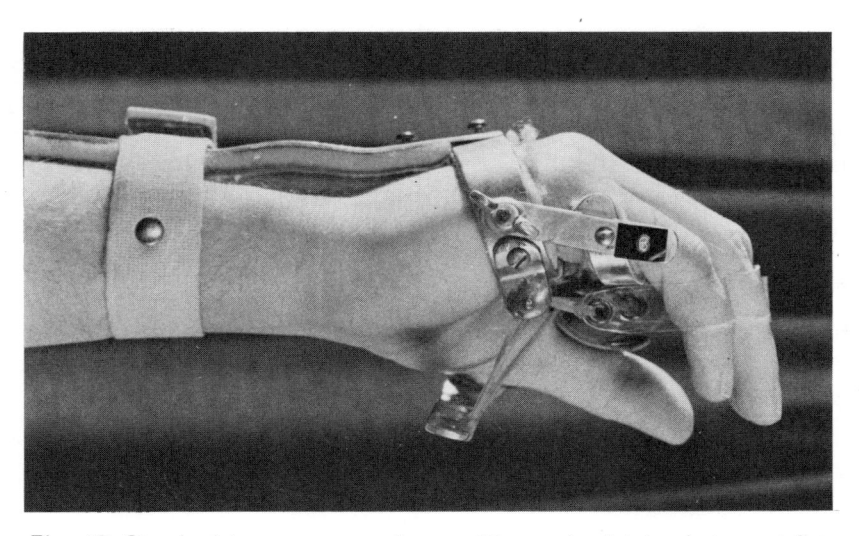

Fig. 48. Standard long opponens brace with proximal interphalangeal flexor assist. Note the offset extensor bar to control ulnar drifting of the fingers.

Functional Dynamic Bracing

This term is given to any hand splint that stabilizes the affected rheumatoid joints, allowing movement in the opposite direction by means of elastic pulls, at the same time. For example, fingers may be held in extension, allowing active flexion of all the finger joints at the same time. Thus these braces have three functions:

1. To stabilize selected joints.
2. To allow active movements at joints that have good voluntary control.
3. To assist or replace paralysed muscles by elastic sprung or motorized elements.

The dynamic braces have the additional advantage of preventing increase of deformity and are of use to promote healing after surgery.

MASTER TEMPLATE METHOD OF SPLINTING

Another method of making either static or dynamic splints is by means of the Master Template method. The material used is called Orthoplast. It is a thermo-plastic material and is relatively inexpensive. The single basic Master Template design makes it possible to make a variety of splints whether fixed or movable. The movable or dynamic types just need the addition of suspension bar slings, hinges or springs.

Method of construction. The pattern (Fig. 49) can be drawn on brown paper or paper towelling. The latter can be dampened for moulding.

(1) Outline the patient's hand on the paper, marking the position of all joints of fingers, hand and wrist.
(2) Draw the pattern over the outline of the hand.
(3) Try the pattern on the patient's hand.
(4) Outline the pattern on a sheet of Orthoplast.
(5) Heat the Orthoplast by one of two methods: (a) a heat gun may be used, heating both sides until a slight impression is obtained by finger pressure, or (b) immersing the Orthoplast for a short time in water brought to boiling point and then simmered. It is easier to use the second method.
(6) Cut the pattern outline.
(7) Fit and mould the splint.
(8) Add extra attachments if required. Rivets or staples can be used.

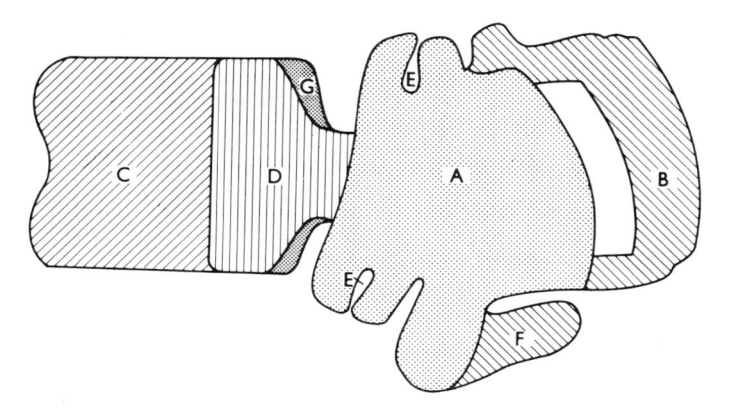

Fig. 49. Basic pattern for master template method of splinting. (a) Main part of hand. Metacarpal phalangeal section should extend midway to the proximal joints of the fingers. The thumb section should extend to the middle of the hypothemar area of the palm. (b) This section should extend to midway past the distal joints towards the ends of the fingers. (c) This section should wrap half-way round the arm. (d) The curves of this section should correspond with the condyles of the ulnar and radius. This area can be increased or decreased to fit the arm. (e) Gussets to facilitate fitting of the splint. (f) Thumb section which can be extended to the distal joint of the thumb. (g) May be cut away, or used as extra reinforcement by turning over the edge.

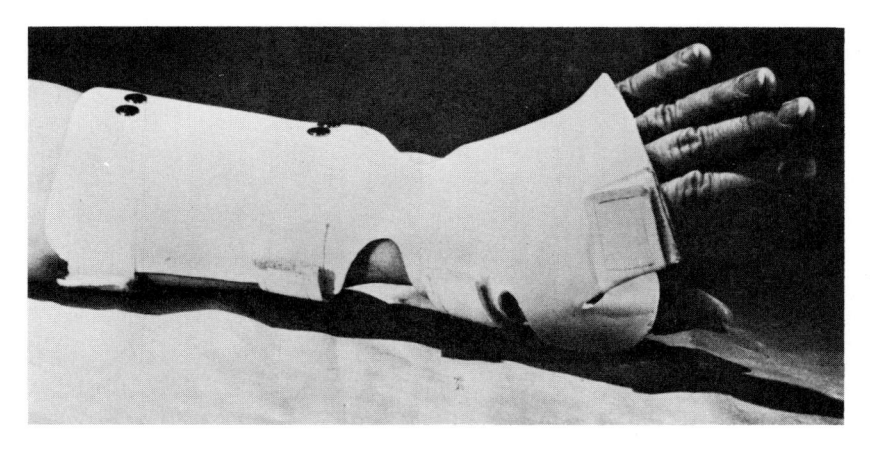

Fig. 50. Extension of wrist and opposition of the thumb.

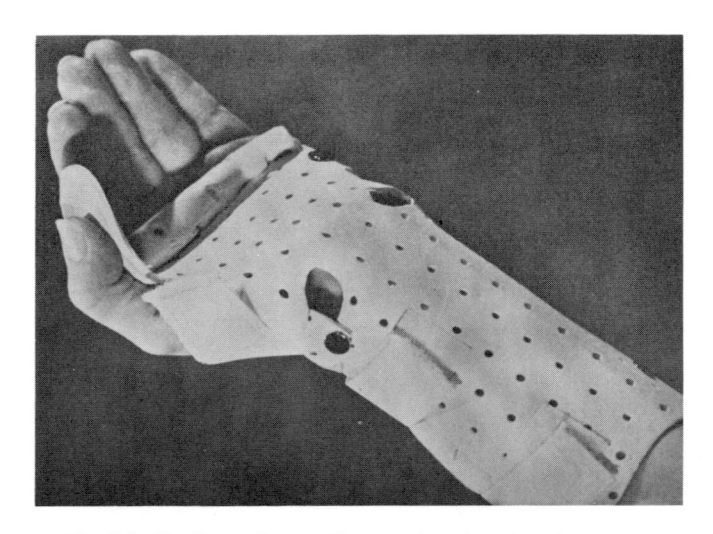

Fig. 51. Similar splint as Fig. 50 showing thumb at rest.

5
Wrist splints

COCK UP SPLINTS

Short Metal Cock Up Splint

These splints can be stocked in varying sizes. They are designed with a ball-like structure which fits into the palm of the hand, and gradually flattens out towards the wrist resembling a shoehorn. The splint (Fig. 52) can be made comfortable by covering it with adhesive felt or foam rubber and bandaged on to the hand and forearm.

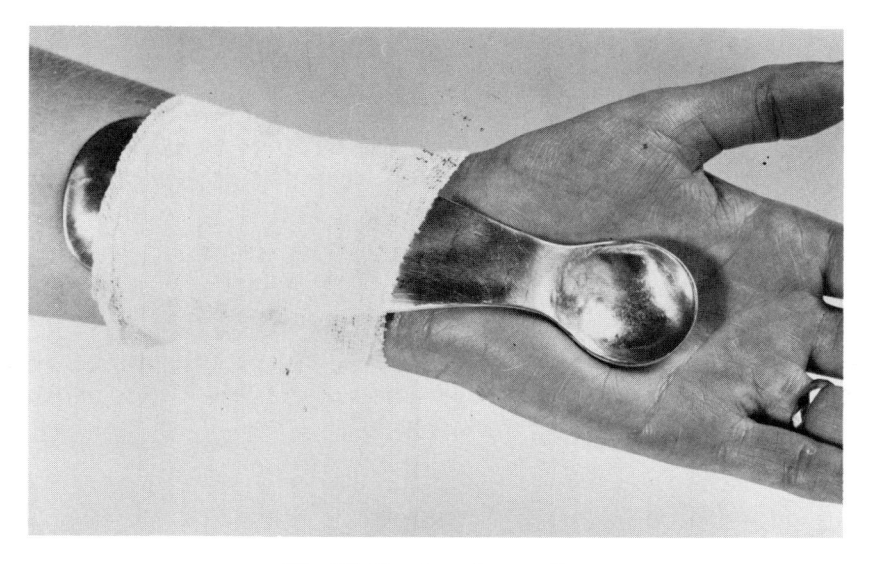

Fig. 52. Short cock up splint.

Long Cock Up Splints

This metal splint (Fig. 53) extends from below the elbow to the tips of the fingers and thumb. It is not often used, due to the necessity to keep all the digits moving, but it has a use in cases of sepsis and as an alternative to plaster after surgery.

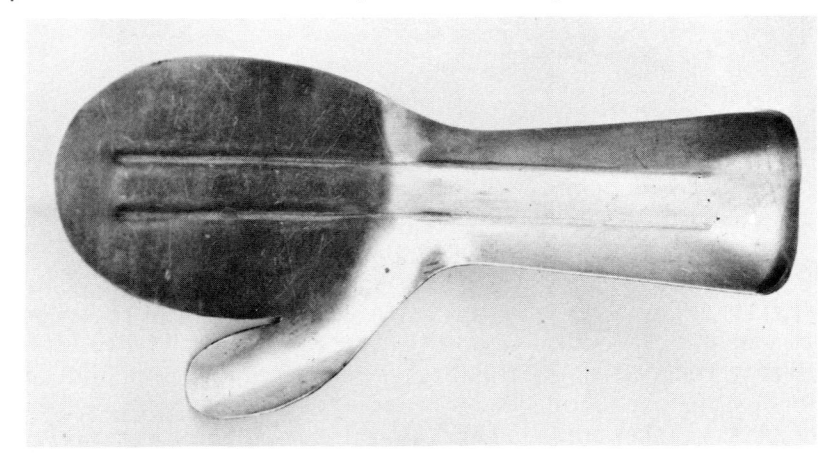

Fig. 53. Long cock up splint.

PALMAR SPLINTS

In some fractures of the metacarpals it is necessary to bandage all the fingers in flexion over a firm sponge, wire pad or even a suitably sized bandage.

WRIST STRAP

A simple leather wrist strap of about 2 in. (5 cm) in depth can be a help to patients with a chronic weakness of the wrist. These patients are usually men with heavy manual jobs.

6
Elbow splints

The elbow joint is possibly the least splinted of all joints.

The Sling or Triangular Bandage

The arm is held at about 90 degrees of flexion. One-half of the bandage is passed behind the affected arm, the other half passes over the front of the arm, and they are joined over the opposite shoulder. The corner by the elbow is firmly pinned to the sling at the back of the elbow. A sling is worn for injuries to the hand, wrist or elbow, or even to the humerus, and the angle at the elbow can be varied. It is also an adjunct to the splinting of the shoulder in cases of severe fracture of the clavicle.

Collar and Cuff

This is used in elbow injuries when it is necessary to have about 45 degrees of flexion at the elbow. It is also used in conjunction with plaster for some types of fracture of the humerus. The collar and cuff (Fig. 54) is made of leather tubes, one longer than the other, through which two lengths of strong (non-elastic) bandage are passed. The bandage through the shorter wrist cuff is joined to that of the longer neck cuff, and the tension is adjusted as required. The tubes can also be made of sewn felt or any other similar material.

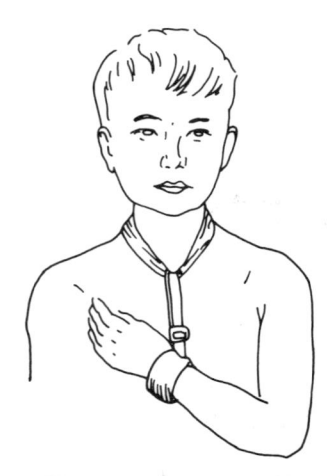

Fig. 54. Collar and cuff.

ARM SPLINTS

The Webbing Sling

A simple 2-in. (5-cm) webbing strap with a fixed loop at one end and a sliding loop at the other end, enables the arm to be held in contact with the chest, the elbow being held at a right angle (Fig. 55). It is useful for injuries of the shoulder and humerus.

Application. The forearm rests in the fixed loop. The strap then passes across the back, over the opposite shoulder and down to the wrist, which lies in the adjustable loop. Thus the arm is kept against the chest wall.

Moulded Leather Elbow Support

The moulded leather arm support is usually a permanent splint and may be used in cases of bone diseases, non-union of fractures and the flail arm. This splint is the same in appearance as the hinged moulded leather elbow splint (Fig. 56) except that the whole area of the arm is block leather, thus eliminating all movement of the elbow joint. The measurements are taken by means of a plaster cast, special attention being paid to prominent bony points. These should be marked by an indelible pencil on the skin so that the mark is

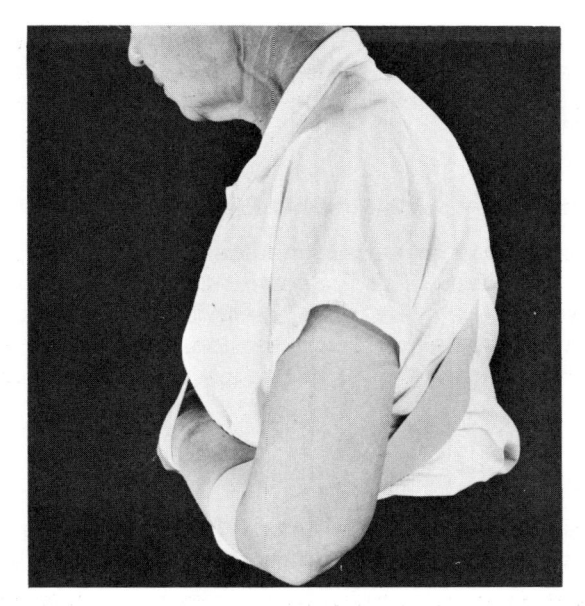

Fig. 55. Webbing arm support. Note the close proximity of the arm and chest.

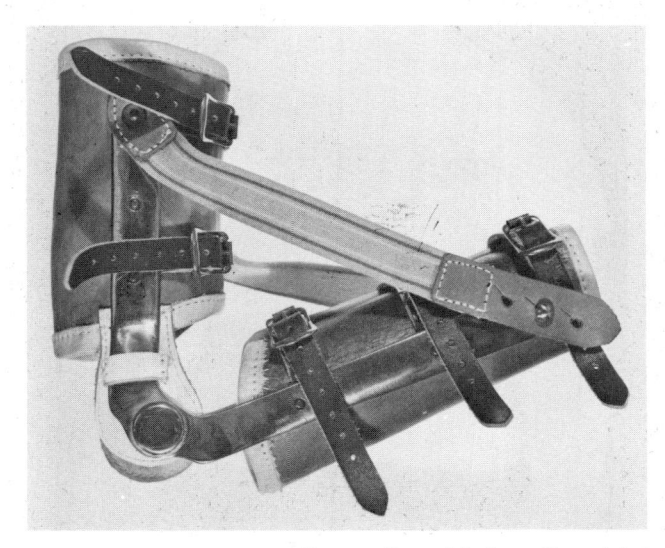

Fig. 56. Moulded leather elbow splint with free elbow joint.

transferred to the plaster. The leather is moulded on to the filled and stripped cast, and when dry, is fitted to the patient, adjusted, notes made on possible alterations, and then sent to the Workshops to be finished.

Moulded Leather Splint, with Movable Elbow Joint

The upper and lower arms have moulded leather bands, but a free joint is used at the elbow. This is a particularly useful splint (Fig. 56) for protection of the joint in haemophiliac patients. It gives protection, yet allows flexion and extension. Special care should be taken to see that the joint does not touch the elbow, and produce bruising.

Clavicle Splint

The clavicle splint (Fig. 57) is used for treating the fractured clavicle, and is designed to keep the shoulders braced in extension,

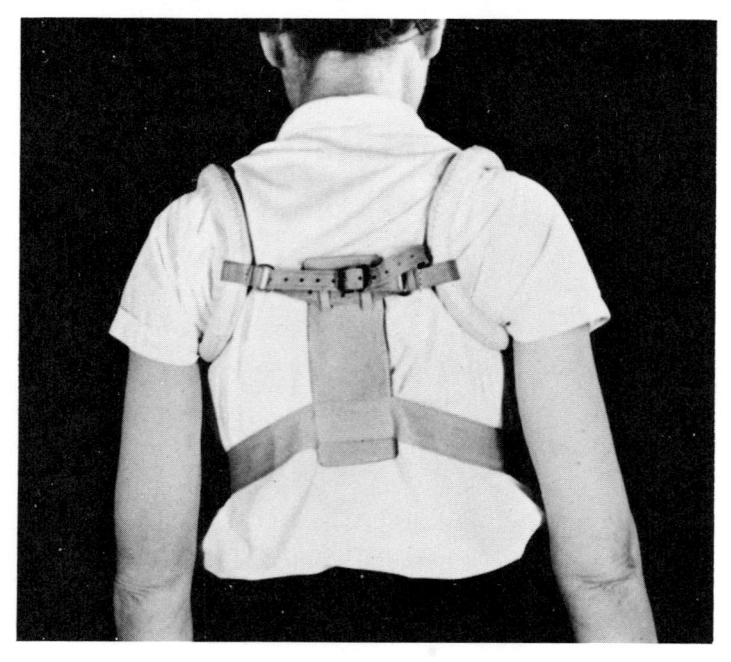

Fig. 57. Clavicle splint.

thus preventing an overlap of the fractured ends which, if allowed, might give rise to a bony prominence—a deformity to be avoided, especially in women. The clavicle splint comprises two circular leather straps with buckle fastenings. These are joined by an adjustable strap across the scapular region of the back and can be pulled quite tight. These splints can be kept in stock in varying sizes. In centres where these splints are not available, the same principle can be carried out using stockinette tubes. Two-inch stockinette padded with wool can encircle both shoulders and should be long enough to be joined in the centre of the back. This type of splintage will probably need to be tightened daily. Triangular bandages can also be used, but this is a more clumsy method. The arm on the side of the fracture may need to be rested in a sling. Occasionally, a pad of cotton wool may be put under the axilla of the affected side.

7
Shoulder splints

Arm Abduction or Aeroplane Splints

These splints (Fig. 58), always an essential for an Orthopaedic Department and usually kept in a selection of sizes, are made of $\frac{5}{16}$ in.-gauge mild steel. The steel framework is covered with leather slings which support the arm, and canvas straps for keeping the splint in position.

Measurements. The following measurements are necessary to enable a well-fitting splint to be applied:

(1) Length (measure the good arm abducted at 90 degrees of flexion) from the centre of spine to point of elbow.
(2) Length from the point of the elbow to the metacarpal phalangeal joints.
(3) Length from the axilla to the iliac crest.
(4) Circumference of the chest.

When fitting the splint it is advisable to have an assistant to hold the affected arm in abduction, so that the splint can be slipped under the arm. The strap to be fastened first, is the one which lies over the opposite shoulder, followed by the other straps encircling the trunk. Usually the lower bar rests on the iliac crest. If this bony point is not palpable, most of the strain is taken by the strap which passes over the sound shoulder. It will usually be found easier to measure the patients sound arm. A bandage may be necessary to keep the arm in position on the splint.

The aeroplane splint was primarily designed for polio cases with paralysis of the deltoid muscle. It is sometimes used in the treatment of a ruptured supra spinatus tendon, after an acrominectomy and a

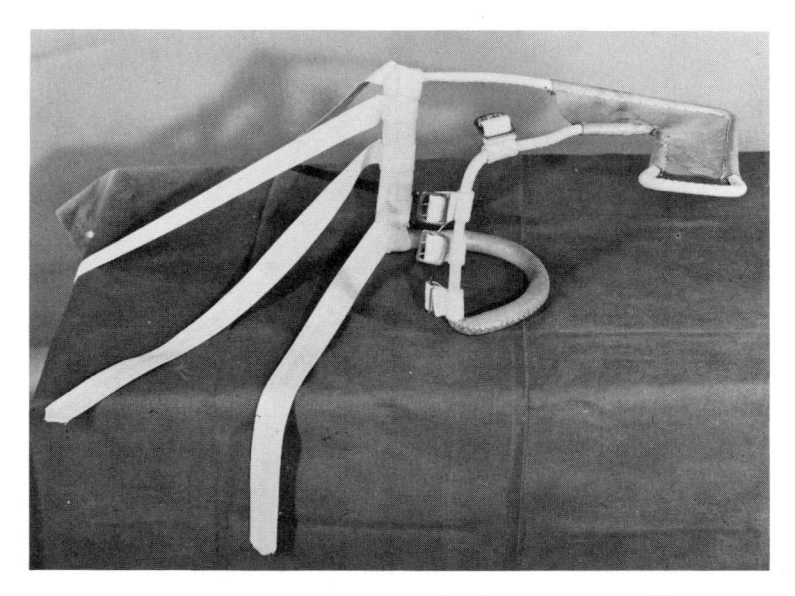

Fig. 58. Aeroplane splint for abduction of the shoulder.

brachial plexus injury. It can be used with physiotherapy, for gradually raising the arm during treatment of a frozen shoulder. Both the arm portion of the splint and the semi-circular trunk portion can be adjusted to the patients requirements. It should be noted that the aeroplane splint does not immobilize the shoulder, it merely rests it in the abducted and slightly flexed position. For immobilization, a thoraco-brachial plaster is required.

Fairbanks Splint

The Fairbanks splint (Fig. 59) is an arm abduction splint designed to treat an Erb's palsy with the characteristic deformity of internal rotation and abduction of the shoulder, extension of the elbow and flexion of the wrist. Consequently the splint rests the shoulder at 10 degrees of abduction and slight flexion, the elbow in 90 degrees flexion, and wrist in neutral position. The splint is made of padded duralumin—as it is usually used for the young rapidly growing baby. Plaster of Paris can be used instead, and renewed at weekly intervals.

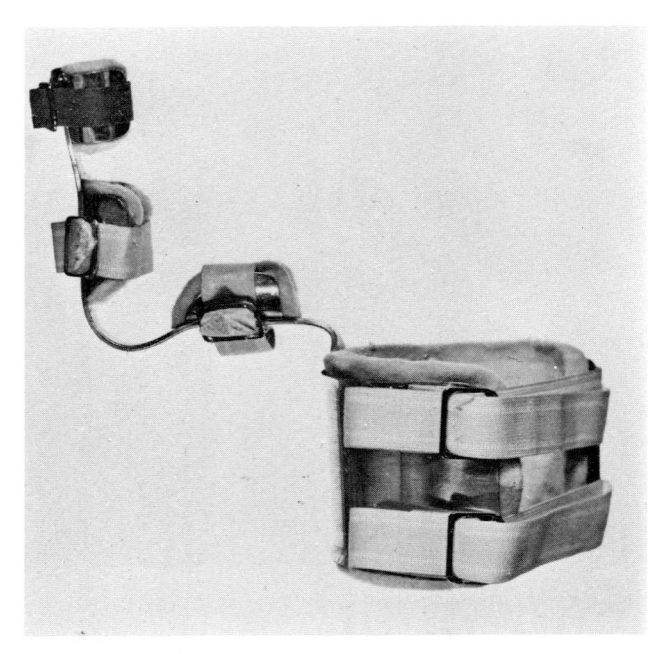

Fig. 59. Fairbanks splint.

The measurements required are the same as for the aeroplane splint (see p. 72).

8
Calipers

THE PRINCIPLE OF WEIGHT RELIEVING

The principle of weight relieving must be understood before the fitting of a caliper, designed to take some of the body weight of the hip and knee joints, can be carried out. Calipers are designed either to give stability to a weak or flail leg, or to relieve a diseased hip or knee joint of some of the body weight. In order to carry out the latter principle, the ischial tuberosity must rest on the ring or tuber hold of the caliper, the weight is then transmitted down the shanks of the caliper to the heel of the patient's shoe, with the patient's own heel being elevated off the ground. There should be one finger's breadth space between the plantar surface of the patient's own heel and the shoe. If preferred, it may be easier to visualize the weight transference the opposite way, that is, from the heel of the patient's shoe, with the heel gap, up the shanks of the caliper to the ring and so to the ischial tuberosity. It is, very important therefore that the caliper fits correctly. The ring must fit under the tuberosity; if it is either too big, or too small, it will not be weight relieving (Fig. 60). The length of the caliper is equally important; if it is too short, the patient's heel will rest right down in the shoe, and the caliper will not be weight relieving.

Some small boys have very small ischial tuberosities, and it is almost impossible to keep the ring, however well fitting, underneath the tuberosity. It will be necessary to make a lozenge shaped ring which may be difficult to apply, but it does keep the ring beneath the tuberosity.

When a caliper is being worn to give stability to a leg, the fit of the ring is not so important, but naturally, a well-fitting ring is to be preferred. The patient's foot rests down in the shoe so that a stability caliper does not have to be as long as a weight-relieving caliper. Needless to say, the fitting of a caliper which has to be a non-weight relieving is very much easier.

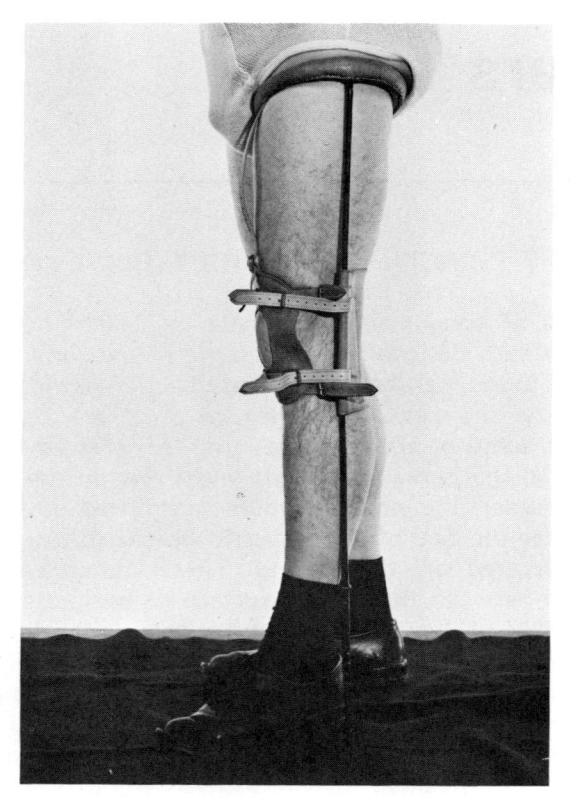

Fig. 60. Weight-relieving calipers.

Ring Caliper

The design of the ring caliper (Fig. 61) is the same whether it is used for weight relieving or to give stability to the leg. The ring is hemi-spherical and tilted downwards on the inner side. It is made of $\frac{1}{2}$-in. round steel, which is covered with grey felt to act as padding, which, in turn, is finally covered with a smooth leather (usually basil leather). The ring is joined at each end of the sphere with the two metal shanks which lie on the medial and lateral sides of the leg, and terminate in adjustable ends. These caliper ends are made so that the upper part is slightly flattened, with four screw holes for length adjustment, and the distal ends have round pegs set at a right angle to fit into the tube set in the patient's shoe.

If the caliper is a weight relieving one, in the growing child, it is very important to see that it remains weight relieving. This is done by lengthening the caliper. The shanks have four corresponding holes at the adjustable ends, and the screws can be removed, the ends moved down, and screws re-applied. There is a $\frac{1}{2}$-in. (1·2-cm) gap between each screw. The knee is kept in position by anterior and posterior knee leathers. The posterior one being a leather sling designed to prevent hyperextension of the knee. The anterior leather sling is

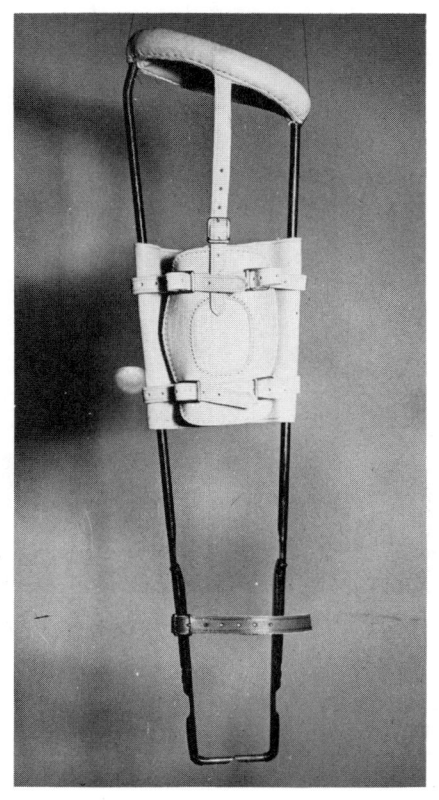

Fig. 61. Ring caliper, showing anterior and posterior knee leathers.

roughly square in shape with a soft central area to cover the bony patella. It has four straps, with either buckle or Velcro fastenings at each corner, which slip round the metal shanks and fasten anteriorly. The anterior knee leather may also have a $\frac{1}{2}$-in. (1·2-cm) strap going from its upper border to the front of the ring. All calipers have a $\frac{1}{2}$-in. (1·2-cm) leather ankle strap which encircles the patient's ankle and prevents the caliper ends from coming out of the heel tube; this can happen when the caliper ends begin to wear.

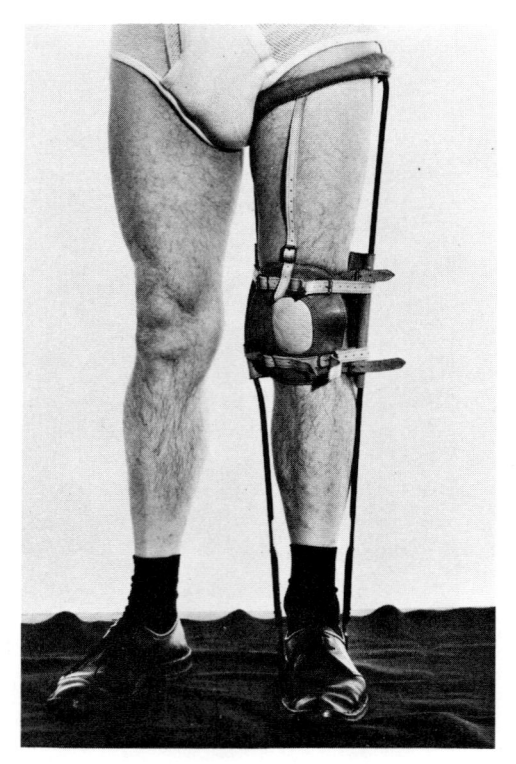

Fig. 62. Ring caliper, showing anterior and posterior knee leathers.

Measurements. Two simple measurements are required, but they need to be carefully taken.

(1) Circumference of the thigh at the highest possible level, with the tape measure held firm and straight.

(2) The length from the ischial tuberosity to the plantar surface of the heel.

It is advisable when measuring the length of a weight-relieving caliper to take the top length measurement well on to the ischial tuberosity in order to get the required extra $\frac{1}{2}$-in. length. If the caliper is being made in a hospital workshops it is advisable to fit the splint before it is finished so that alterations can be made more easily. This is known as fitting 'in the rough', and in these cases the ring is not covered with leather, the metal is unpolished, and the straps are temporary.

A very light caliper may be required if the patient is light in weight, and the good leg is strong. Duralumin may be used, but it must be remembered that this metal alloy, though very light is also very brittle, and may not stand up to excessive strain. The standard metal used is double sheer steel. Very often a $\frac{1}{2}$-in. temporary raise on the sole and heel of the opposite shoe is necessary. This raise helps the patient to carry the leg straight through, thus stopping the affected leg from being swung outward when walking.

Knock Knee Straps

Many patients need a knock knee strap instead of the front and back knee leathers. The knock knee strap is made of very soft leather and is fastened to the outer side of the caliper, exerting a pull on the knee to the outer side, and so helping to prevent a valgus deformity of the knee.

Band Topped Caliper

A band topped caliper (Fig. 63) is designed to give protection to a knee joint or stability to a leg. It may be used in cases of haemophilia for protection of the vulnerable knee joint, for stability for the spastic patient, or bilaterally with or without a pelvic band, for a child with spina bifida. In these cases the ring is either not tolerated, could cause bruising, or is an encumbrance for the child without bladder control.

Measurements. The band at the top of the caliper is made of thick leather which is not moulded and so does not need a plaster cast. This type of caliper is chosen for the haemophilia patient. It always

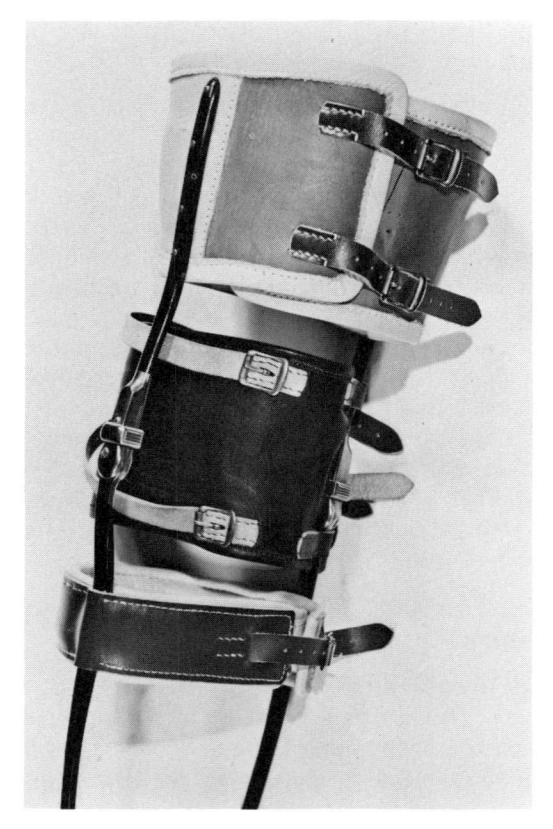

Fig. 63. Band topped caliper, showing knock knee straps.

has a knee joint to encourage knee movement, but it can be kept locked when necessary. The measurements taken (by means of a tracing of the leg) for the correct alignment, are the length from just below the ischial tuberosity to the plantar surface of the heel, the length from the knee joint to the plantar surface of the heel, and the following circumferences:

- (1) The top of the thigh.
- (2) Mid thigh.
- (3) Above the knee.
- (4) Level with the knee joint.
- (5) Below the knee.

(6) Mid calf.
(7) Above the ankle joint.
(8) The ankle joint.

The patient's leg should rest on a hard surface, such as a wooden table or fracture board. The tracing paper, preferably a strip of brown paper, is laid under the leg and on top of the hard surface, and should extend from the lower buttocks to include the heel. All these measurements should be very carefully carried out, correct alignment for haemophiliacs and the spina bifida children being especially important. The facility of bruising in haemophiliacs, and the tendency for sores due to lack of sensation in spina bifida must be remembered. Fitting a caliper with a knee joint needs extra care. It is important to see that the caliper joint is opposite the patient's knee joint, and that there is about $\frac{3}{8}$ in. (9 mm) space between the metal and the patient's leg on either side, which is maintained when the knee is flexed. In the case of bilateral calipers, careful fitting is necessary to see that the medial surfaces of the knee joints do not knock one another. It is very often necessary to fit these calipers with knock knee straps. The type of lock generally used is the ring lock.

Patten Ended Caliper—or Thomas' Walking Splint

The patten ended caliper (Fig. 64) should always be a weight relieving splint, and is accompanied by a compensatory patten worn on the shoe of the sound side. It is one of the splints for resting a Perthe's disease of the hip. The principle of weight relieving is perhaps easier to understand than in the ring caliper. The patten ended caliper, as its name suggests, ends in a patten instead of pegs fitting into the heel tube. Thus the weight is transmitted from the ischial tuberosity to the ring of the caliper down the shanks, to the patten, with the patient's leg slung between the shanks, and the foot some 1 to 2 in. (2·5 to 5 cm) above the patten. On no account should the foot rest on the patten. If it should do so, the splint would no longer be weight relieving. The patten is 2 to 3 in. (5 to 7·5 cm) in depth, while that on the good side is $\frac{5}{8}$ in. (15 mm) deeper, allowing the affected leg to be swung straight through, rather than swinging outwards when walking. The measurements are the same as for a ring caliper, the depth of the patten being decided by the instrument makers, and being proportionate to the total length.

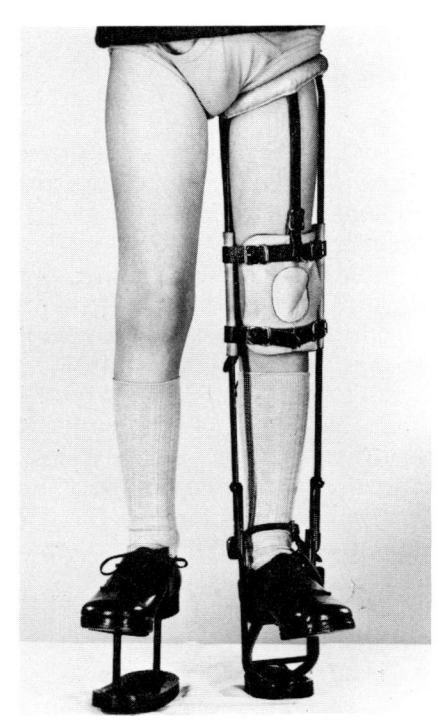

Fig. 64. Patient wearing patten ended caliper.

The caliper is a comparatively heavy splint, being made of double sheer steel, the patten and additions to the shoe, adding to the weight. Usually a webbing sling is attached to the front and back of the ring, this passes over the opposite shoulder and fastens low in front. The patten is usually blocked with leather and covered with rubber to prevent slipping. The patten on the caliper is adjustable, and the caliper can be lengthened in the same way as in a ring caliper.

Shoe alteration. In theory it is not necessary for a shoe to be worn, and, in fact, in the early stages of rehabilitation it may be left off, in many cases children have difficulty in keeping their foot in the shoe. However, a strong pair of lace-ups is advocated for the attachment of the patten on the good side, and for the front and back check stops to be fitted to the shoe of the caliper (Fig. 65). These stops slide on either side of the shanks and prevent the foot from pointing downwards and causing non-weight relieving.

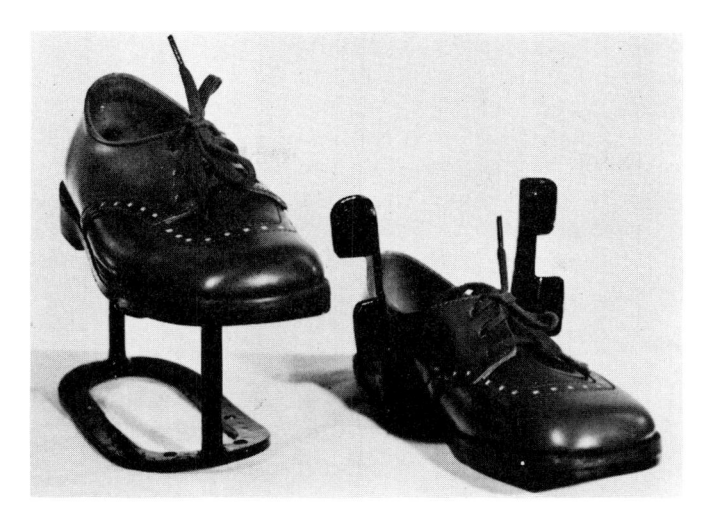

Fig. 65. Shoes with compensatory pattern (left) and front and back check stops (right).

Bucket Topped Caliper

The bucket topped caliper (Fig. 66) can be weight relieving or not as required. It should always be weight relieving when used after a patient has had a pseudarthrosis of the hip. When used for a patient

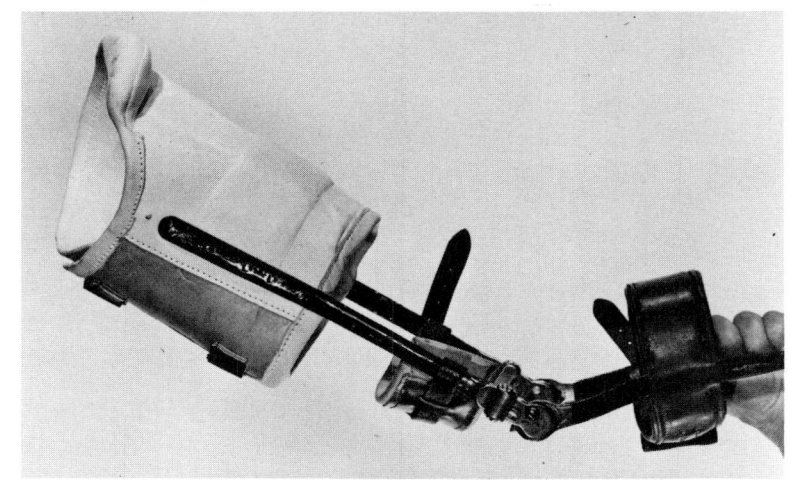

Fig. 66. Bucket topped caliper, showing ischeal tuberosity bearing hold.

with a weak or paralysed leg it is not, as a rule, weight relieving, though some polio patients like to 'sit' on the ischial hold. Generally speaking, adults do not tolerate ring calipers, and so are provided with bucket calipers. Children can usually adapt to most things. If a patient has worn a ring caliper all his life, he will probably prefer to continue with one. Young men in the accident wards, with slow union of fractures, may be given a ring caliper to wear for a time. Of course, a bucket top caliper takes longer to make and is more expensive. Any splint with a joint is heavier, and more costly.

Measurements. The leather in a bucket topped caliper is moulded and to obtain the correct linear measurements a plaster cast is advisable. This is a procedure which the elderly patient who has had surgery, finds troublesome, therefore, she should be told before-hand what is about to take place.

Preparation of the patient. The plaster cast may be taken pre- or post-operatively, usually the latter. All traction, etc., should be removed from the patient. A small, firm pillow or soft sandbag should be placed under the buttock of the affected hip. It is preferable to have the patient lying on a hard table, but it may be necessary to keep the patient on her bed, in which case the bed should be well protected with polythene sheeting.

(1) Using a wet indelible pencil, the ischial tuberosity should be marked on the patient's skin, as also the position of the knee joint. If the knee joint is difficult to palpate, the patella or its lower border could be outlined. It is sometimes difficult to locate accurately the ischial tuberosity, particularly in the obese patient. To help the instrument maker the following measurements can be taken: (a) the length of the leg, ischial tuberosity–plantar surface heel; and (b) knee joint–plantar surface heel.

Note: If the knee is valgus, then a knock knee strap will be necessary.

Most adult patients are given a knee joint unless they have a stiff knee.

(2) The patient's leg is covered with a stockinette stocking. It should extend from the toes to 2 to in. (5 to 7·5 cm) above the top of the thigh, to protect the perineum from plaster, and to cover the ischial tuberosity.

(3) A length of cast wire is laid down the outer side of the full length of the leg.
(4) A bucket of warm water should be ready, and a trolley containing 6-in. (15-cm) Gypsona bandages, a small plaster slab, consisting of four layers, 6 x 8 in. (15 x 20 cm), an indelible pencil and a sharp cobbler's knife.
(5) The patient's leg is carefully held with the hip in flexion and abduction, 5 degrees of flexion of the knee. The plaster is applied evenly to include the ischial tuberosity and heel. The small slab should be laid over the ischial tuberosity, and incorporated in the plaster.
(6) When the plaster has set (only sufficient need be applied to maintain the shape when it is removed), the area of the length of wire which lies between the stockinette and plaster, is marked with a series of horizontal lines, the wire is gently pulled, and the plaster is cut with the knife against the wire, until it is open the full length. The stockinette is cut with a pair of Elastoplast scissors and the whole cast gently removed from the patient's leg (Fig. 67).

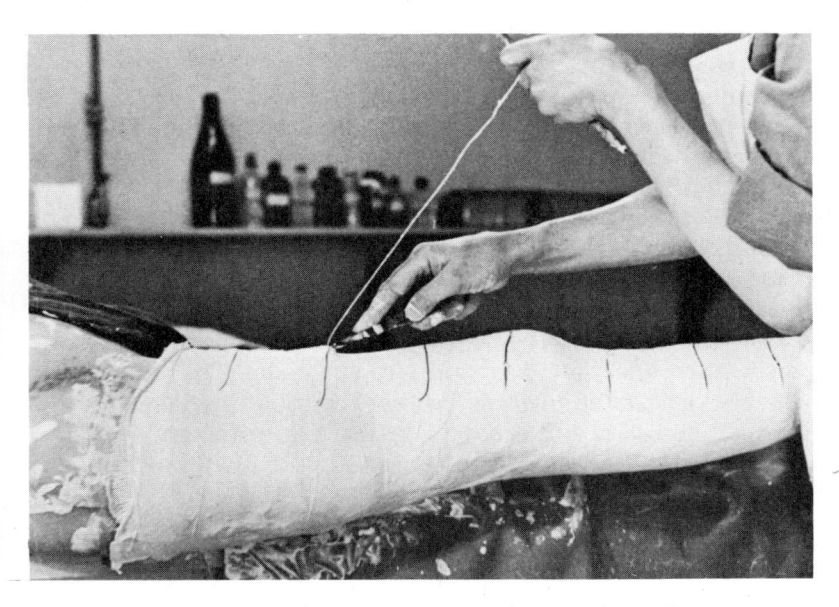

Fig. 67. Removing the plaster cast for a bucket caliper.

(7) While the patient is being washed and returned to her traction, the cast is joined with plaster bandages, so that the series of horizontal lines are in apposition with one another. The cast is now ready to be filled and sent to the workshops.

Fitting of the caliper. At the time of taking the cast, a comfortable pair of shoes should be sent to the workshops to have the heel tubed, preferably a pair with a broad heel and laces. Difficulty can be experienced in obtaining a suitable pair of ladies shoes, as so many only wear slip-on shoes (casual or court shoes). If this is so it may be necessary to add a retaining heel strap so that the shoe does not slip off the patient's foot, which may happen if the caliper is truly weight relieving.

Patients with pseudarthrosis of the hip generally have a shortening of that limb of 1 to 2 in. (2·5 to 5 cm). A temporary raise of the necessary height to equalize the limbs should be applied to the shoe. In order to make walking easier the depth of the raise may be reduced by $\frac{1}{2}$ in. (1·2 cm). The caliper is ready for a fitting when the bucket is attached to the shanks, and temporary straps have been applied. The shoe should also be raised and tubed. The leather is not lined or polished, so the fitting is 'in the rough'.

Points to remember when fitting the caliper
  (1) Patient must have the principle of weight relieving explained. It may, otherwise be difficult to understand why the heel should *not* rest right down in the shoe.
  (2) The patient must sit up in bed with both legs straight. The affected leg should be lifted up and laid in the caliper, the shoe having been first put on but not laced. Note whether the leg is externally rotated and correct if possible. If the leg is externally rotated (it may well be as a result of pseudarthrosis) then the first correction to the caliper will be to have the bucket rotated inwards, so that the tuber hold is *under* the ischial tuberosity and not digging into the perineum.
  (3) Note the level of the caliper knee joint—it should be opposite the patient's knee joint.
  (4) Note the amount of flexion of the patient's knee, the caliper may have to be altered accordingly.
  (5) Take care to see that the total alignment is correct, so that none of the metal touches the leg. It is necessary to flex the

knee, with the caliper on, as there often is a change in alignment. The ankle region is also a vulnerable part.

(6) Check especially the length of the caliper, it must be long enough to make it weight relieving. This can really only satisfactorily be done by standing the patient and slipping a finger underneath the patients heel. This is difficult for the patient, he should be supported on either side and encouraged to stand up straight.

(7) If there has to be an alteration made in the length of the caliper, it should be decided whether the change should be above or below the knee joint.

(8) Mark on the bucket top, the level of the overlap of the leather, so that the straps can be fixed in the correct place. The straps are usually of the Velcro type, unless the patient particularly wants the buckle fastenings. Velcro straps have the disadvantage of sticking to clothing, particularly woollens, but they are considered easier to manage.

Unless a knock knee strap is required, the patients knee is free to allow unimpeded flexion. There is, however, a strong leather strap above the knee, below the bucket. The ankle strap is also used. The caliper is finished when the fitting has been accurately carried out. The finished caliper should be comfortable, the bucket lined, the tuber hold padded, and the metal polished. When sitting down the patient needs to slide the ring locks down, so that the caliper flexes, and conversely they need to be pulled up over the hinge to obtain extension on standing.

NON-WEIGHT-RELIEVING BUCKET CALIPERS

This is a bucket caliper which stabilizes the weak leg and very often does not have a tuber hold, but merely a slight thickening at the inner side of the posterior edge of the bucket (Fig. 68). The measurements and casting are the same as for the previous caliper. The fitting is easier, in that there is not likely to be a rotational deformity of the hip, and the patient's foot can rest right down in the shoe.

The joint of the caliper is an automatic one and slightly more costly to make. If the patient has a weak or paralysed leg, it will be necessary for him to manually straighten it before standing. While

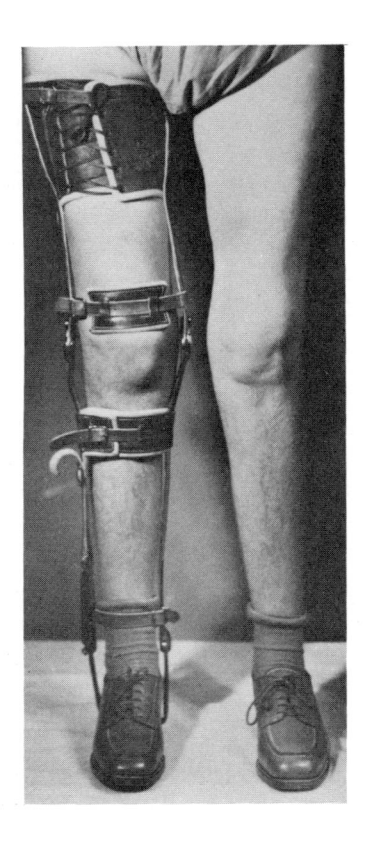

Fig. 68. A patient wearing a non-weight-relieving bucket caliper. Note the ankle joints and flat sockets.

the leg is being straightened, the knee joints lock in extension (Fig. 69). Before sitting down the patient usually pulls on the hoop which lies at the back of the knee, this flexes the caliper and knee. There can be a strap of either strong elastic or leather extending from the hoop to the back of the bucket, and the patient may give this a slight pull before sitting.

A completely flail leg will have below knee modifications to the caliper, flat ends, to prevent plantar flexion, a joint to allow ankle movement, and a side spring to help dorsiflexion. Most weak and flail legs need knock knee straps.

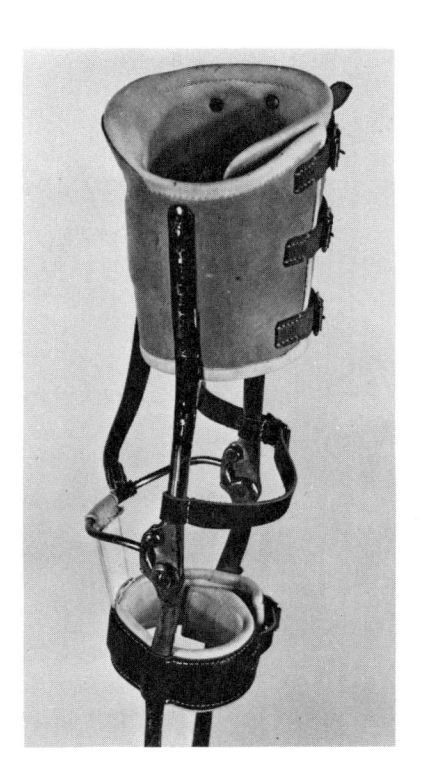

Fig. 69. Non-weight-relieving bucket caliper, showing the automatic or bar lock knee joint and no tuber hold.

Shortening. Polio patients, especially if they contracted the disease as a child, will almost certainly have some shortening of the leg, which may be as much as 4 to 5 in. (10 to 12·5 cm). It is essential that the amount of shortening is added on to the length measurement, otherwise, when the caliper is fitted it will be found to be short. The raise on the shoe is usually cork (see Fig. 109), and is inserted between the uppers and sole and heel, so that the heel tube is *below* the raise, hence the need to add the shortening to the total length of the caliper. In cases of pseudarthrosis when the shortening is apt to vary, the raise is a temporary one fixed below the heel tube.

BUCKET CALIPERS

A non-weight-relieving caliper may end in a leather heel cap (Fig. 70) which fits inside the shoe. This means that the patient's shoes need not be tubed, but there may be some difficulty in obtaining a suitable shoe.

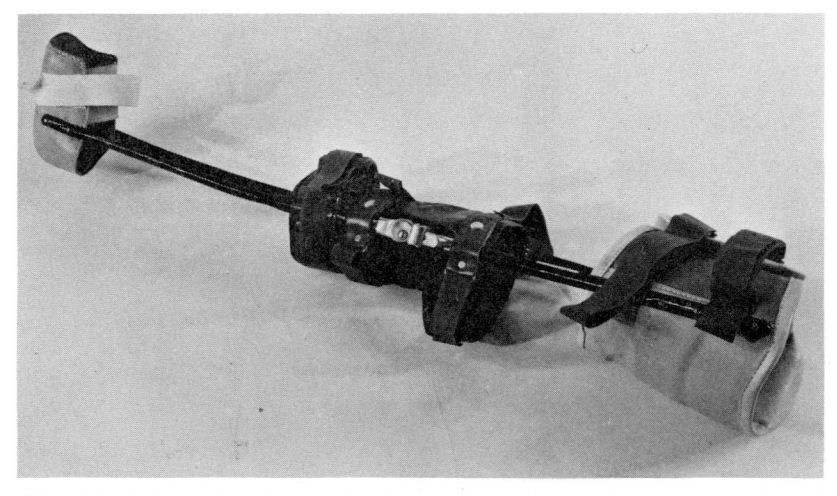

Fig. 70. Caliper showing leather heel cap and knock knee strap with Velcro fastenings.

CALIPER FOR THE PATIENT WITH RHEUMATOID ARTHRITIS

This is normally the band topped variety which is very light and made of duralumin with ring locks. These ring locks are attached to small side springs, which, in turn, are attached to a hoop which lies across the front of the thigh. The hoop is added to enable the rheumatoid patient with affected fingers and hips to flex the knee without bending forward or managing the small ring locks. However, it has a big disadvantage: if the patient cannot manage to manipulate the knee, he will not be able to put the caliper on unaided, so he is dependent on the caliper being put on for him. The measurements may be a cast or tracing. A cast is preferable if there is much deformity present.

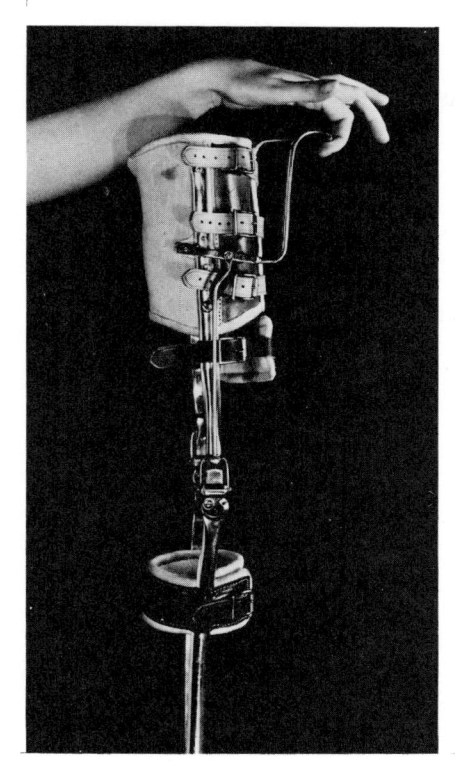

Fig. 71. Caliper showing knee locking hand grip.

The Stanmore Concealed Caliper

Mr W. H. Tuck of the Royal National Orthopaedic Hospital has developed an unobtrusive caliper of good cosmetic appearance. It is hygienic, light in weight and suitable for the polio patient with flail leg (Fig. 72). The bucket is made of Ortholen, a high density polyethylene. This is a strong material with some spring in it. It is moulded on to the cast at a temperature of 190°C. The Ortholen is used for the posterior lower leg and foot. It extends from the tibial condyles, narrows behind the calf and extends under the foot to the metatarsal heads. This prevents foot drop and allows the use of ordinary shoes.

The intervening area between the bucket and tibial condyles has stainless steel shanks with knee joints. If the patient has a

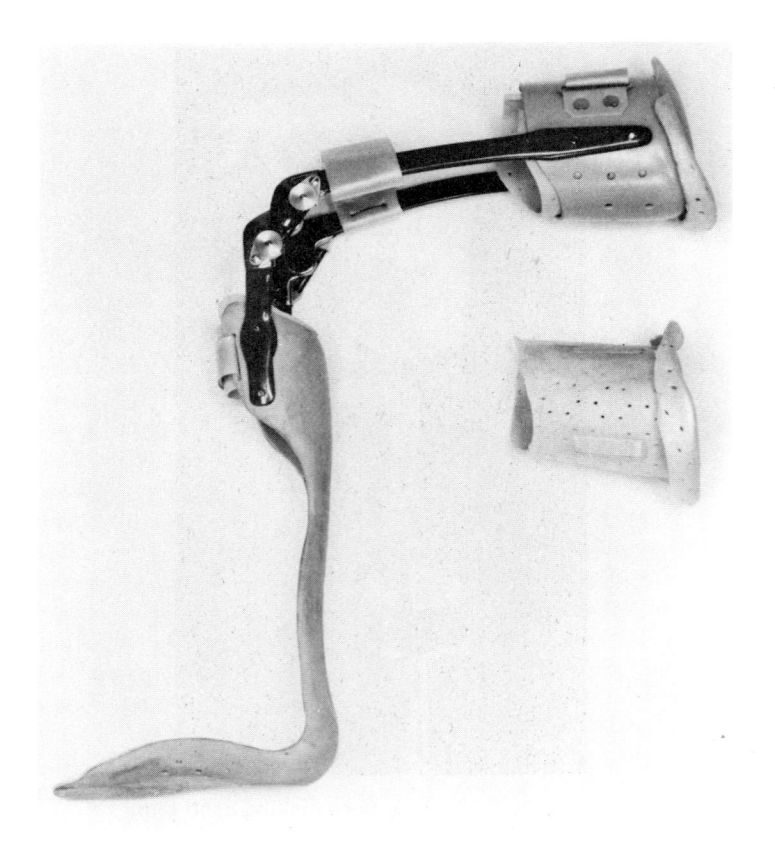

Fig. 72. Stanmore concealed caliper.

hyperextending knee, Otto Bock's free joint, with limitation of hyperextension can be used. The weight of the caliper is $2\frac{1}{2}$ lb. (1 kg). A stainless steel bar lock joint can be used for the patient who cannot walk without a knee locking device. Features of this splint are a detachable plastazote lining $\frac{1}{4}$ in. (6 mm) thick for the inside of the bucket, and an artificial muscle for the calf, made of plastazote to match the opposite leg. This is mainly for female patients. Several calf linings can be supplied to the patient and they are, of course, easily washed. The straps on the bucket, above the knee, and on the drop foot appliance, are made of very thin Ortholen, with plastazote pads. These are fixed with Velcro webbing to the main Ortholen.

Measurements. These are taken by a complete plaster of the leg, to include the foot, which should be at right angles.

Combination of Double Calipers and Pelvic Band

Patients who require double calipers for stability of the legs may also need assistance in keeping the trunk erect. The gluteal muscles in these cases fail to work sufficiently, and the hip flexors take over. The added stability can be achieved by the addition of hip joints which lie opposite the patient's hip joints and are incorporated in a metal strip which extends from the outer side of the top of the caliper to the pelvic band. These joints may either be of simple flexion and extension, or have the addition of abduction and adduction joints. The dual joints are particularly useful if a spastic child is to be splinted. The flexion joints facilitate sitting, the extension can be limited for standing with sufficient play for walking. The adduction is usually limited to prevent the scissor gait with a small amount of abduction allowed.

The usual measurements are required for the calipers but the following additional measurements are necessary:

(1) The length from the great trochanter to hip joint.
(2) The length from the hip joint to the waist.
(3) The circumference of the waist.

Sometimes the rings of the calipers are split to make for easier application. The pelvic band should be hinged or be sufficiently malleable to open easily. If a pelvic band is not sufficient to keep the trunk erect, a moulded leather or polythene jacket may be used instead. The jacket is joined to the calipers in the same way. Casts of the trunk would be necessary.

9
Spina bifida cystica

This condition arising more frequently due to improved surgery after birth, is one that is presenting problems of satisfactory splintage which is still in the experimental stage. The children have either a total paralysis from waist downwards, or some muscle reflex action not controllable by the patient. If there are some strong muscles working they will eventually prove deforming. These children need to have their joints stabilized so that they can keep the erect position.

The Shrewsbury Splint

This appliance (Fig. 73) is designed to give stability to the lower back, hips, knees and feet at the same time allowing a swivel gait. The large foot pieces allow the centre of gravity to fall within the area of the foot pieces, extremely important when the mobile patient has been made into a comparatively rigid structure.

Description of the splint. Padded leather covered metal bands encircle the chest and pelvis. They are joined laterally by metal shanks which extend to the patient's heels. There are leather thigh and below knee bands. Open toed laced bootees form part of the splint. On the soles horizontal ball bearing devices are fixed so that the foot plates can rotate on the splint. The foot pieces are very large to begin with, to prevent the child falling over, but they can be reduced in size later.

Locomotion (Fig. 74) is obtained by one foot moving forward in the arc of a circle, the centre of which is below the other foot. A return spring is provided, so that the internally rotated footplate resumes its normal position in the air. When the child transfers its weight to footplate A, B rotates forward, the weight is transferred to B and footplate A returns to the normal position, and, in turn, travels forward. This splint is also known as the 'Clicking Splint'.

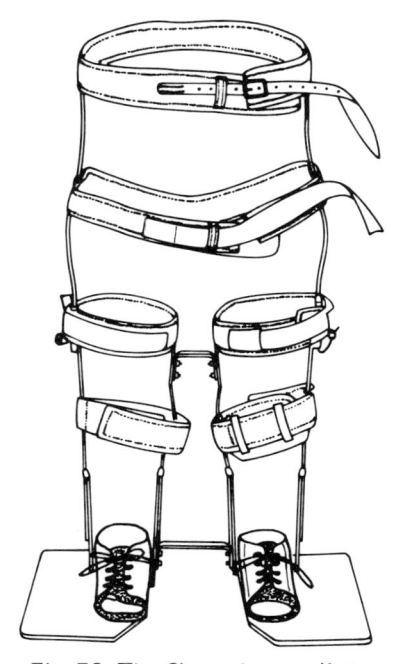

Fig. 73. The Shrewsbury splint.

Measurements. The measurements are simple, the difficult part is teaching the child this form of locomotion. The measurements are as follows:

(1) Circumference of the chest below nipple line.
(2) Circumference of the pelvis.
(3) Circumference of the lower thigh.
(4) Circumference of the leg at fibular head level.
(5) Length down the outer side of the trunk from below the nipple line to the plantar surface of the heel.
(6) Length down the inner side of the leg from 1 in. (2·5 cm) below the perineum to the plantar surface of the heel.

If preferred a tracing can be taken of the legs and pelvic bulge. Ordinary shoe measurements also need to be taken.

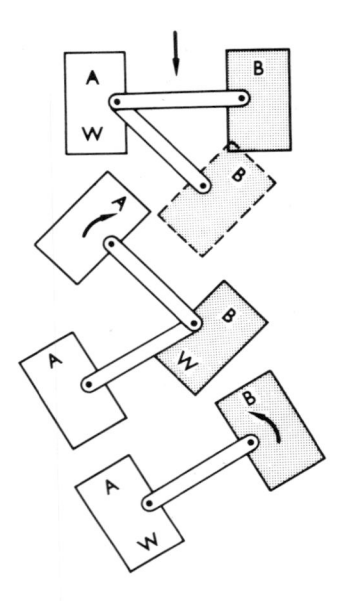

Fig. 74. Diagram illustrating transferance of weight.

The Sheffield Calipers and Brace

The Sheffield calipers and brace (Fig. 76) are designed to give movement at the hips and stability to the trunk. The hip joints are of the double locking variety. The patient is able to walk with 20 degrees of flexion, and 150 degrees of extension, combined with a small range of abduction and adduction. The ability of the child to adduct and abduct the hip enables him to transfer his weight by a rocking movement from side to side within the brace, thus facilitating walking.

The brace is of the skeletal variety, but a feature is the low slung transverse sacral bar to prevent the child from tilting his pelvis and developing a hip flexion contracture. The transverse sacral bar may be divided into two, with a tongue on either side curving downwards to lie over the glutei (they are joined by an adjustable leather strap). In either case the pressure of a scar or tumour in patients with meningoceles is avoided. Occasionally it is necessary to have a broad chest piece to prevent the child from leaning forward. Weak abdominal muscles may make the addition of a corset necessary.

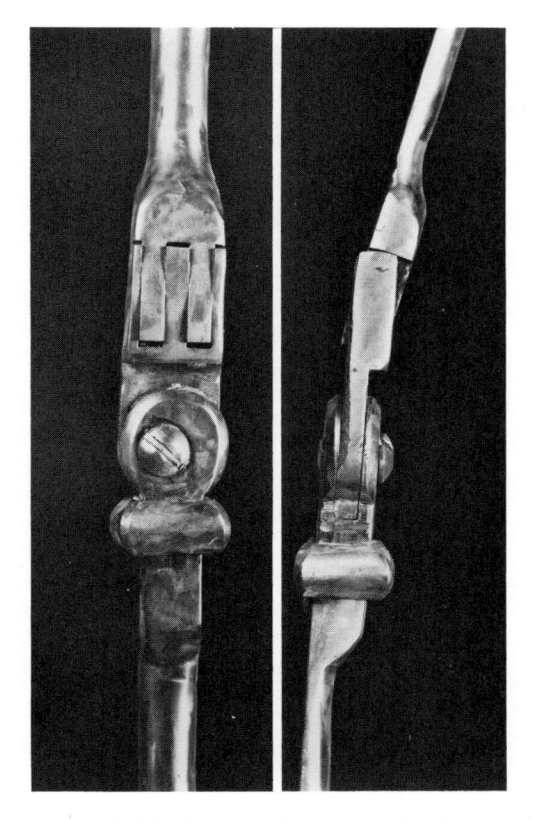

Fig. 75. Sharrard joints, showing flexion, extension and abduction and adduction lock.

Carshalton Calipers

The purpose of the calipers is to give support where there is weakness, and allow movement when possible. The apparatus should be cosmetically acceptable. The Carshalton Caliper (Fig. 77) has straight legs, hip joints and corset top. The hip joints are made to allow full range of flexion, 10 degrees of extension, 5 to 15 degrees of abduction and 5 degrees of adduction. The cuff top is connected to the waist band by a leather strap which can be unfastened at the top when the child sits. This strap can be removed when the child can control knife-jacking at the hips. The corset is made of soft

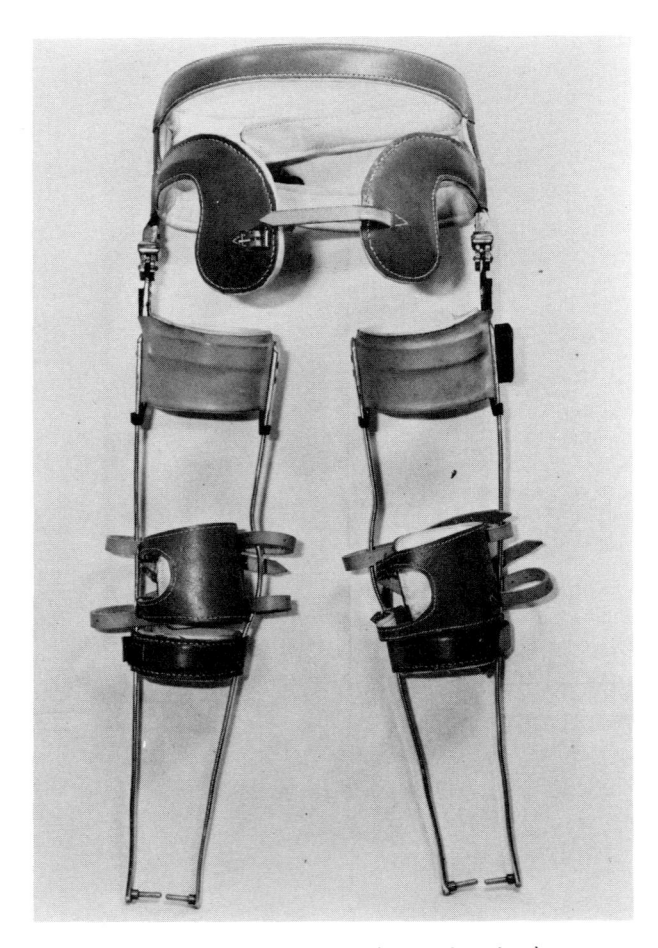

Fig. 76. Sheffield brace (posterior view).

leather with Velcro fastenings. The upper and lower posterior bands of the corset can be shaped to accommodate a kyphos. The lower band should lie at the maximum convexity of the gluteal region.

Lower Limb Bracing with Mobile Jacket

The older patient with paraplegia may find locomotion easier by keeping the legs and hips stable, but the trunk support moderately

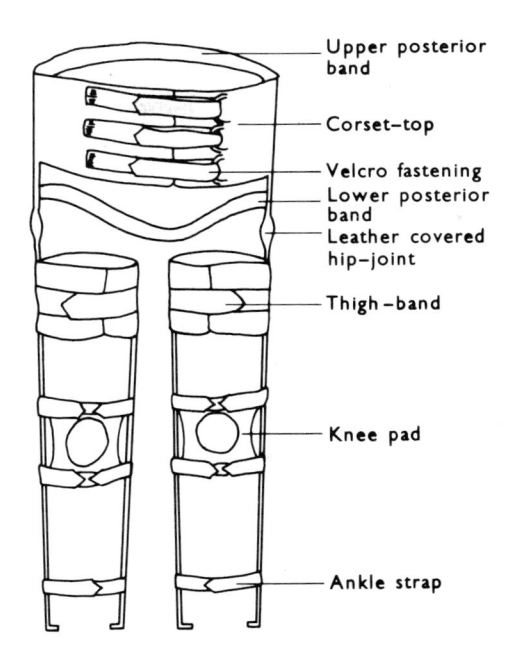

Fig. 77. Diagram of Carshalton calipers for spina bifida.

mobile. This is obtained by full leg calipers set in relationship to each other and to the trunk. The hip joint complex may be of two kinds. There may be simple joints to allow limited flexion and extension with a simple axis in one plane. This enables the patient to sit, and the joints can be self locking. The moderately mobile trunk band is light in weight. Rotation of the trunk is obtained by cables above the hip joints across the back. This allows the body to rotate round a vetical axis. There may be an additional limited abduction joint. Above and below this joint lie two short horizontal bars. The two posterior cables are attached to these bars.

Double Calipers with Pelvic Band, Hip joints and Gluteal Elastic Straps

This useful combination (Fig. 80) allows for rigid legs and mobile area above the hip joints. The ring tops are split, that is, they open

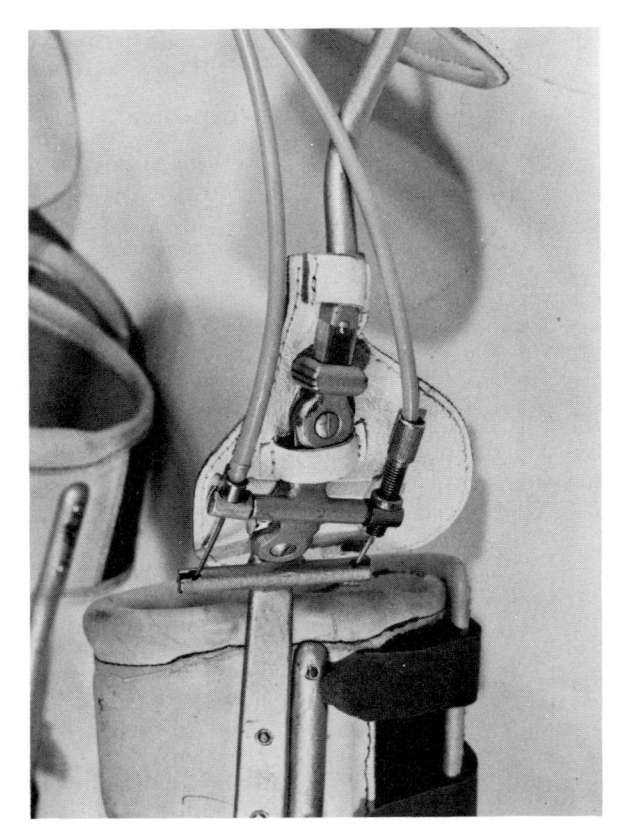

Fig. 78. The flexion and extension joint, and below the abduction joint with the cable fixtures.

anteriorly for easy application. The hip joints are of the ring lock variety and allow for easy sitting adjustment. The back of the rings are joined to the pelvic bands by strong 1-in. (2·5-cm) wide elastic which is detachable at the top. This gives stability in the gluteal region when the child stands and at the same time allows the child to sit. There should be a soft leather sling at the back of the thighs, and the usual anterior and posterior knee leathers. The calipers should end in adjustable flat ends to prevent dropped feet, and the shoes should be tubed accordingly.

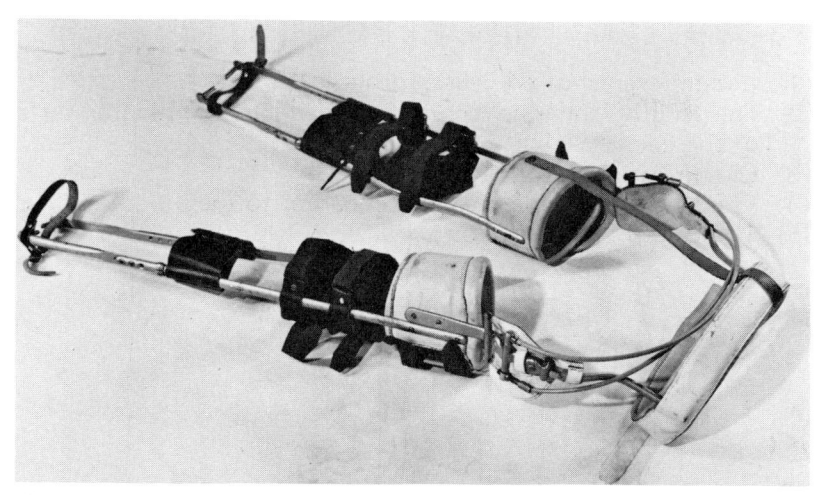

Fig. 79. Lower limb bracing showing cables to allow rotation of the trunk.

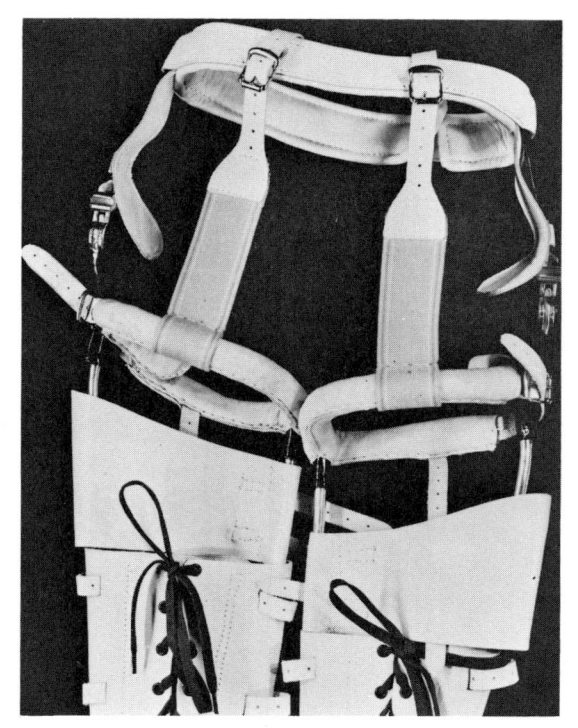

Fig. 80. Double calipers with hip joints and elastic hip bands.

Measurements. The measurements are as follows:

(1) Circumference of the legs at groin level.
(2) The length from the ischial tuberosity to the plantar surface of the heels.
(3) Circumference of the waist.
(4) The length from the greater trochanter to the hip joint.
(5) The length from hip joint to waist.

10
Perthe's disease

Snyder Sling

The simplest form of resting the hip joint in the case of Perthe's disease of the hip is the Snyder sling. This maintains the hip joint in flexion, abduction, and slight internal rotation. The patient wears a leather strap $1\frac{1}{2}$ in. (4 cm) wide round the waist. Attached to this strap is one that passes over the shoulder on the opposite side of the affected hip. Also attached to the waist band is a narrower leather strap that passes through a metal hook fixed to the back of the heel of the patient's shoe. This is the important part of the appliance, as the tension controls the degree of flexion and rotation of the hip. The top ends of this strap are attached: (1) laterally and anteriorly to the waist band, and (2) centrally posterior to the waist band. The sling has a buckle fastening. The positioning of the top ends of the sling, control the rotation required. The patient's knee should be at a right angle, with the foot well off the ground. Axillary crutches are usually used.

Measurements. The measurements required are:

(1) The circumference of the waist.
(2) The length (with the knee flexed at 90 degrees) from the waist band to the top of the back of the heel.
(3) The length from the front of the waist band laterally over the opposite shoulder to the back of the waist band laterally.

All the slings are adjustable. Very often the patient is given a night splint which maintains slight flexion and internal rotation of the hip. The important point is that the patient should be non-weight bearing on the affected side.

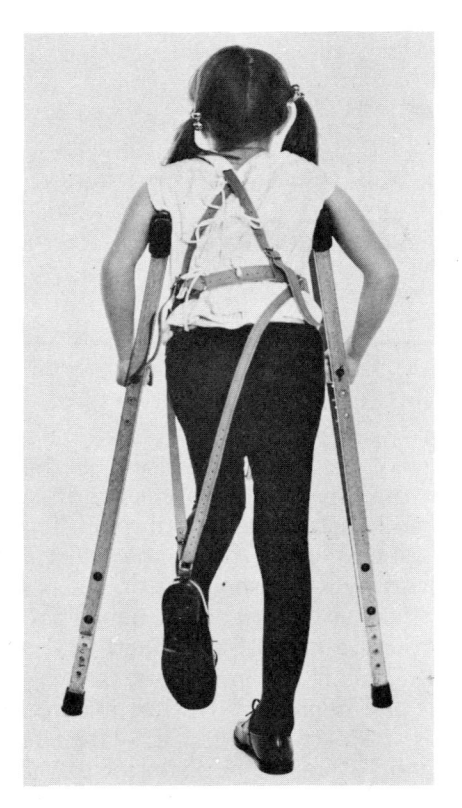

Fig. 81. Posterior view of a patient wearing a Snyder sling.

The Birmingham Containment Hip Splint

This splint, also known as the Harrison splint (Fig. 82) is designed to hold the hip in flexion, abduction and internal rotation in cases of Perthe's disease of the hip. It is a strong splint and maintains the required position without difficulty. It allows the patient to attend school and lead a fairly normal life. The construction of the splint takes time and a plaster cast is required. The cast should be taken with the child resting on a hip stand and the required position of flexion, abduction and internal rotation of the hip being manually held. The cast should extend from below the nipple line to just beyond the heel of the patient's foot, flexion of the knee at 90

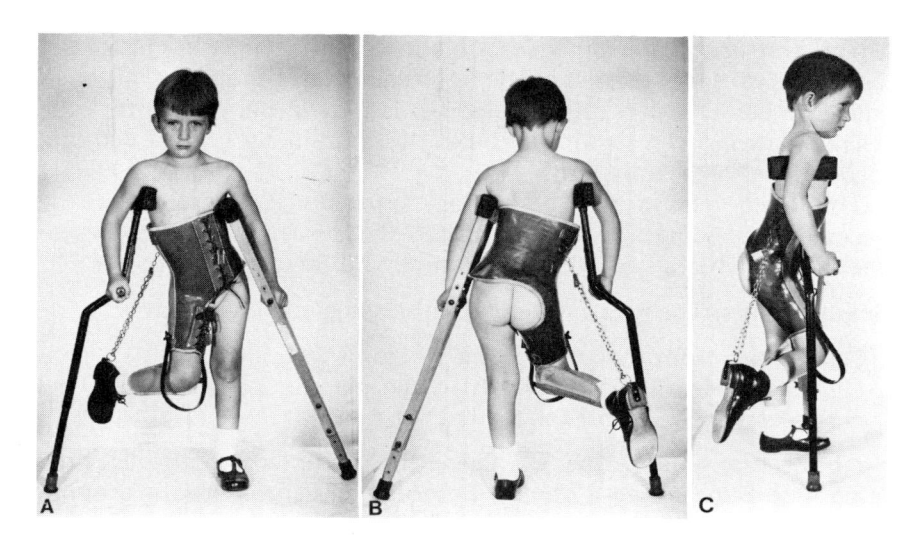

Fig. 82. The Birmingham containment hip splint, sometimes known as the Harrison splint. (a) Front view, note the staggered crutch. (b) Posterior view, note the internal rotation of the hip. (c) Side view.

degrees being maintained. If it is only possible to extend the cast to the knee, then a measurement should be taken from the knee joint to the plantar surface of the heel. The main part of the splint, that is the trunk and hip portion can be made of either moulded leather or polythene.

For a description of the splint, we will assume it is made of moulded leather. The trunk portion extends to the nipple line on the normal side to maintain sufficient hip abduction. The thigh portion is strengthened by a reinforced metal strut. Laces, straps and buckles, or Velcro fastenings, are used to close the trunk and hip portion. Laces, though tedious to fasten, maintain the closest contact.

The knee is kept in flexion by the addition of a suspensory chain attached to the lateral side of the upper portion of the trunk to the hook on the back of the heel of the child's shoe. This chain also helps to maintain internal rotation of the hip.

An important part of the appliance is a removable knee stirrup. This takes the weight when the patient is kneeling and prevents transmission of compression to the hips. It is made of tempered steel and is screwed to the thigh piece by a nut and bolt. It should bear an internal rotation flange to maintain internal rotation of the hip. This stirrup and flange are removed at night. A plaster night splint should then be worn to maintain the internal rotation on the affected side—the below knee splint being joined by a bar to control the desired position. This splint enforces the containment of the femoral head within the acetabulum.

The child uses a pair of axillary crutches. The crutch of the affected side being a staggered crutch. It is made of 2·2-cm drawn steel tubing which is bowed to accommodate the abduction.

Measurements. The measurements of the staggered crutch are:

(1) Length from the axilla to the hip joint (grip).
(2) Length from the hip joint to the plantar surface of the heel plus 1 in. (2·5 cm) for the heel of the shoe.

At the grip, the crutch is angled, the abducted length of crutch being 4 to 5 in. (10 to 12·5 cm) before it straightens to the ground.

HIP SPLINTS

Moulded Leather Hip Support

This splint is used where plaster is not desired, usually in cases of sepsis. A plaster cast is required, the patient lying on a hip stand or orthopaedic table of the Hawley or Charnley variety. It extends from the lower ribs to above the knee on the affected side. The patient is unable to sit properly, so it is important to make sure when fitting the patient, that there is sufficient freedom above the thigh on the good side, so that the hip can be properly flexed to allow partial sitting.

Polythene Hip Support

The polythene hip splint is an alternative method to the leather hip support. It is easier to keep clean and lighter in weight. The measurements are by means of a plaster cast as above.

Spiral Splint

The spiral splint (Fig. 83) is designed to control either internal or external rotation of the hip in the small child. It is particularly useful for the child with persistant fetal alignment, when the child fails to

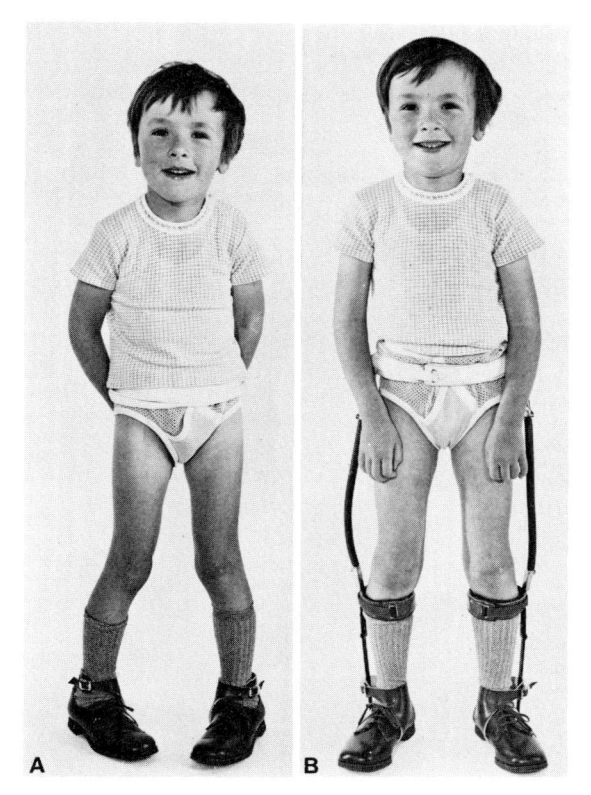

Fig. 83. (a) Child showing internal rotation of the hips due to persistent fetal alignment. (b) The same child wearing the spiral splint, showing the correction of the internal rotation of the hips.

correct with growth, the internal rotation of the hips. The splint has a pelvic band with a free hip joint which allows flexion and extension. The joints are attached to a $\frac{5}{16}$ in. (7·5 mm) five-layer flexible spring known as a shafting wire. This flexible spring wire extends from the greater trochanter to the outer sides of the calf bands which head the double below knee irons. Toe raising springs can be attached to the fronts of the below knee irons if necessary. The direction of the coils of the spring wire is from above downwards and *outwards.* The tension of the wire coils is controlled by a small key which tightens the spring wire at its base, and so the tightened length of the spring wire turns the hip outwards. It is a light and easy splint to wear. If the opposite position is required, i.e. external rotation of the hips, then the direction of the spring coiled wire is reversed, the direction being from above, downwards and *inwards*.

Measurements. The following measurements are taken:

(1) Circumference of the waist.
(2) Length from the waist to the greater trochanter.
(3) The length from the greater trochanter to the level of fibular head.
(4) Circumference of the leg at the level of the fibular head.
(5) Length from the fibular head to the plantar surface of the heel.

11
Congenitally dislocated hip

Congenital dislocation of the hip (C.D.H.) is now frequently diagnosed soon after birth, and the baby can be splinted at once. The mother is able to nurse the baby at home, but it should attend the hospital at regular intervals for splint adjustment and renewal. Splints are usually worn for 2 to 6 months. The splints are made in graded sizes and should be kept in stock so that one can be supplied immediately it is required.

Forrester-Brown C.D.H. Splint

This is made of moderately malleable padded metal bars with a nylon sling between (see Fig. 85). The sling rests under the baby's pelvis, the bars extend down to the feet and are abducted at the level of the gluteal fold. A large metal hoop goes over the front of the baby to facilitate nappy changing. The legs are bandaged to the bars and should be re-bandaged at weekly intervals. At each change the bars are increasingly abducted, until the maximum abduction of comfort is obtained, usually under 190 degrees. A short bandage can be applied round the trunk and splint, which the mother is allowed to remove for washing purposes. A spare sling should be supplied. With full abduction of the legs some difficulty may be experienced with fitting the baby into cots and prams.

S. Von Rosen Splint

This very convenient splint (see Figs 84 and 85) is made of strips of malleable aluminium covered with rubber or waterproof plastic material over protective padding. The malleable portions fold over

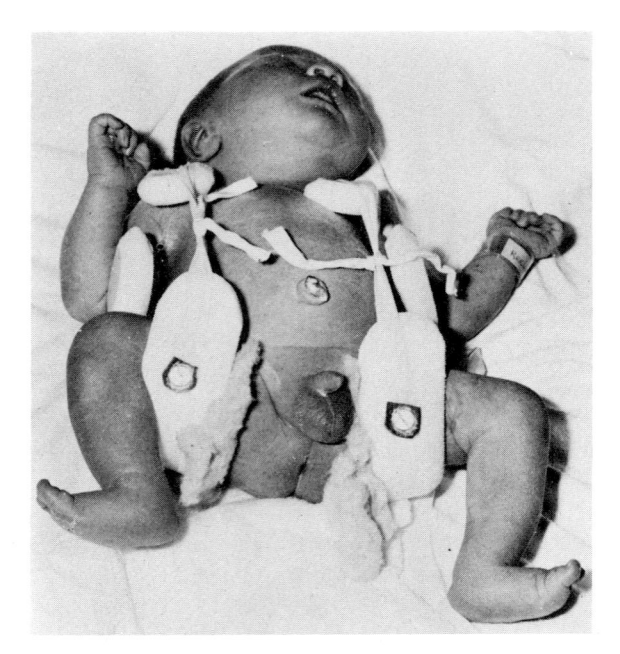

Fig. 84. A baby wearing a Von Rosen splint.

the shoulders for about 2 in. (5 cm), and close in on either side to prevent excessive movement. The lower important malleable sections enclose the upper thighs so that the legs are held in full abduction, the knees remaining flexed. The baby can easily be washed, but the mother must not open the thigh portions of the splints. Hygiene is very important. The baby need not get sore if the skin is kept in good condition and is kept dry. It is easy to apply a thick nappy which should be rectangular and fastened on either side. The baby can be clothed in the normal way and it is hardly noticeable.

Dennis Browne C.D.H. Splint

This splint (Fig. 85) carries out the same principles as the previous splints, viz. wide abduction of the hip. This is obtained by bilateral encircling bands for the thighs. These bands are well padded and covered with a washable plastic material, and joined by an adjustable metal band which lies behind the buttocks. This band, in turn, has a canvas strap joining another canvas strap which encircles the waist.

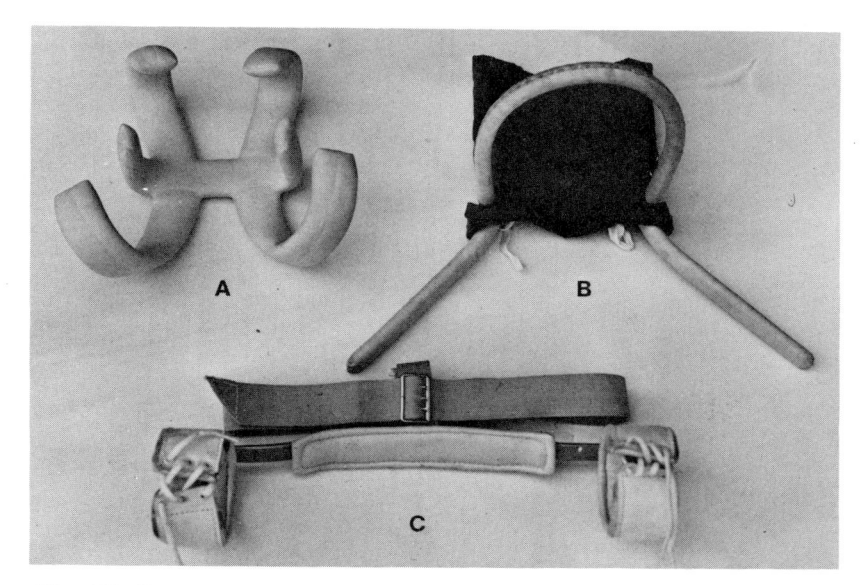

Fig. 85. Photograph showing: (a) Von Rosen C.D.H. splint; (b) Forrester-Browne C.D.H. splint; and (c) Denis Browne C.D.H. splint.

The Dennis Browne splint was designed for older children and can be worn during walking. The gait is difficult, one leg being held well off the ground while the opposite foot is plantargrade. The best way for a child to get around is on a tricycle.

Barlow Cruciform C.D.H. Splint

This splint is made of two padded aluminium strips 22 in. (56 cm) long which are covered with leather or a washable plastic material (Fig. 86). They are riveted together 9 in. (23 cm) from the top. There is a canvas strap which passes through the tops of the strips and fastens in front just below the shoulders. The tops ends of the strips are folded over the shoulders. The lower ends wrap round the upper thighs thus maintaining full abduction of the hips.

The Craig Adjustable Splint

This is a tubular shaped splint made of plastic material with soft foam rubber edges (Fig. 87). It maintains the hips in 90 degrees of

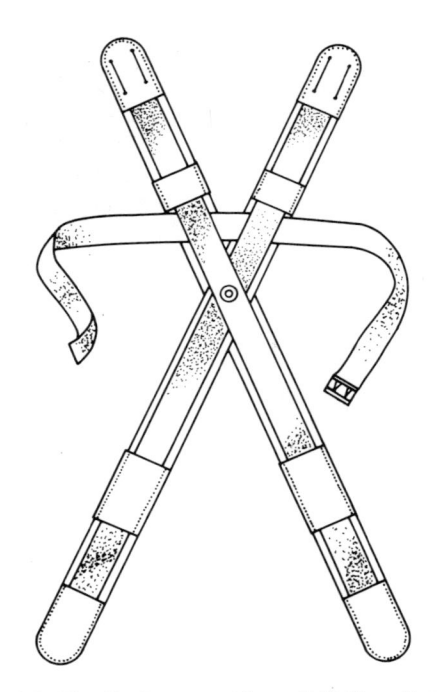

Fig. 86. The Barlow cruciform C.D.H. splint.

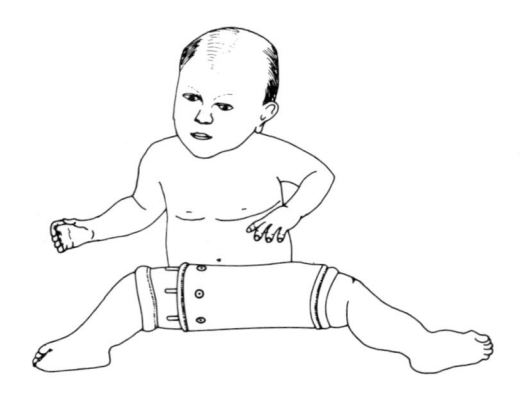

Fig. 87. The Craig adjustable splint.

abduction and flexion. It has the advantage of keeping a nappy in position without pins, the splint being worn outside the nappy. It is adjustable in that one tube overlaps another and so that it can be drawn apart to increase abduction and keep pace with growth.

Double Nappies

For a simple subluxation or suspicion of one, double nappies may be sufficient. They should be folded in rectangles and fastened at the sides.

12
Knee splints

Girdlestone Mermaid Splint

This night splint (Fig. 88) is designed for the child with genu valgum or knock knees. It is used generally in the age range of 2 to 6 years. This postural condition is often combined with valgus feet. The splint is ordered when there is an intermalleolar space of 3 in. (7·5 cm) or more, and is always combined with $\frac{3}{16}$-in. (4·5-mm) wedge heels on the inner sides. These help to relieve the strain on the inner borders of the feet and knees, and tip the feet slightly over to the outer side. The splint is composed to two duralumin gutter splints, wider at one end, joined down the posterior centres so that the legs lie on either side of the gutters. The splint is lined with $\frac{3}{8}$-in. (9-mm) adhesive felt and three webbing straps on either side keep the splint in position.

Application. It is important that the mother is given full instructions on the application of the splint. The child should lie with legs straight, the patellas facing upwards, that is, there should be **no** external rotation. The legs are then drawn into the gutters and the three straps fastened. It will be noticed that the largest gap is between the leg and splint at the ankle region, thus the lowest strap where there is most tension should be fastened first, followed by the other two. It is advisable to instruct the mother to wind a bandage from the top of the splint downwards to include the foot. This helps prevent the child from undoing the straps and protects the sheets from the buckles. After a few days when the child has got used to the splint, a small pad of cotton wool should be placed between the knees and splint. This helps to push the knees outwards while still keeping the ankles together. If the splint is worn regularly, 2 to 4

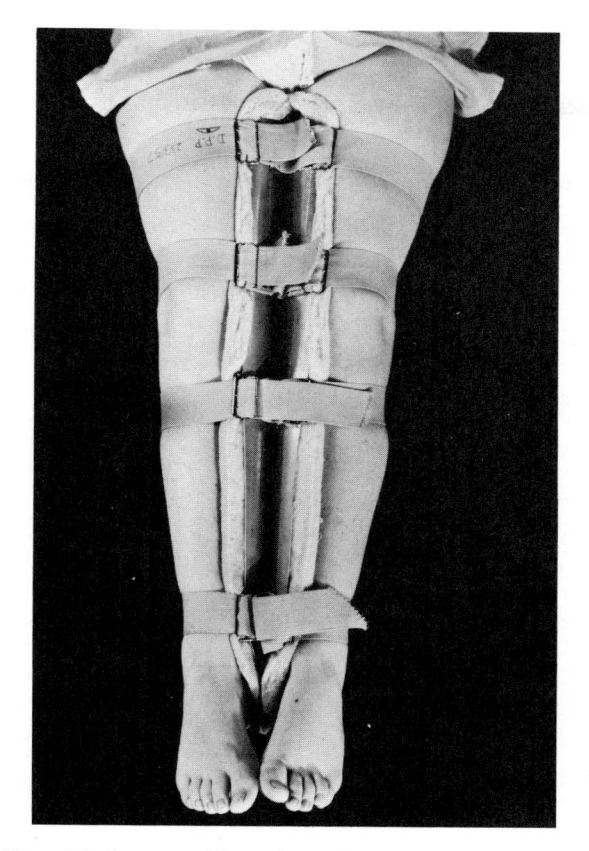

Fig. 88. The Girdlestone Mermaid splint. First application before the insertion of wool pads between the insides of the knees and the splints. Note the patellas are facing straight up.

months will be long enough. On no account should it be worn after the deformity is corrected. The measurement is the length of the leg 1 in. (2·5 cm) below the perineum to the plantar surface of the heel.

Adapted Mermaid Splints for Bow Legs

Occasionally this splint can be adapted for the opposite deformity, generally the child is given extra vitamins and rest for a time each day off his legs, but in cases of obstinate bow legs it may be worn for a longer time. The construction of the splint is the same as for knock knees, but the position of the straps is different. At the point of maximum convexity of the bowing, a wide padded strap is fixed, with the other straps to keep the splint in position. The wool padding is not necessary, but the bandaging is advisable.

Measurements. The following measurements should be taken:
(1) The length of the leg 1 in. (2·5 cm) below the perineum to the plantar surface of the heel.
(2) The length 1 in. (2·5 cm) below the perineum to the point of the maximum convexity of the bowing.

Moulded Leather Knee Support

Patients with an arthritic knee, especially those unable to undergo surgery, can have their leg rested in a moulded leather knee support. It is a comfortable splint, but like all rigid knee supports it is apt to be inconvenient when the patient is sitting.

A plaster cast is taken of the whole leg to include the foot. The splint is reinforced on either side with duralumin which extends to the tubed heel of the patient's shoe. This prevents the splint from slipping down. If the leg is shapely with well developed calf muscles, it might be possible to omit the metal extensions, as the shape of the leg would prevent the downward slipping of the splint. The leatherwork finishes about 2 in. (5 cm) above the ankle. Fastenings are either Velcro or external lacing from the bottom to the top of

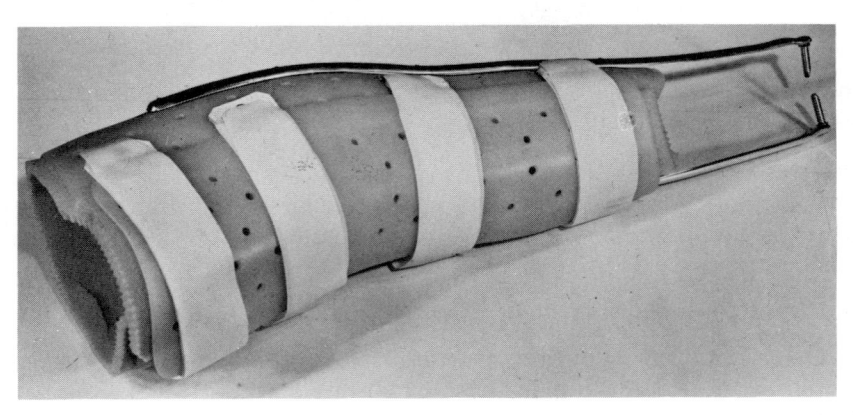

Fig. 89. Polythene knee support. Note the metal shanks to fit into the heel tube, thus preventing the splint from slipping down.

the splint. This ensures the best fitting splint, but is often difficult for the patients to fasten if they have difficulty in bending forwards. This splint may also be made in polythene lined with foam rubber (Fig. 89). It is usually made in posterior and anterior sections, as the polythene is difficult to open if it is in one piece. A plaster cast of the leg is needed.

Howard Marsh Knee Cage

This splint (Fig. 90) comprises padded leather-covered metal thigh and calf bands with padded leather anterior above and below knee

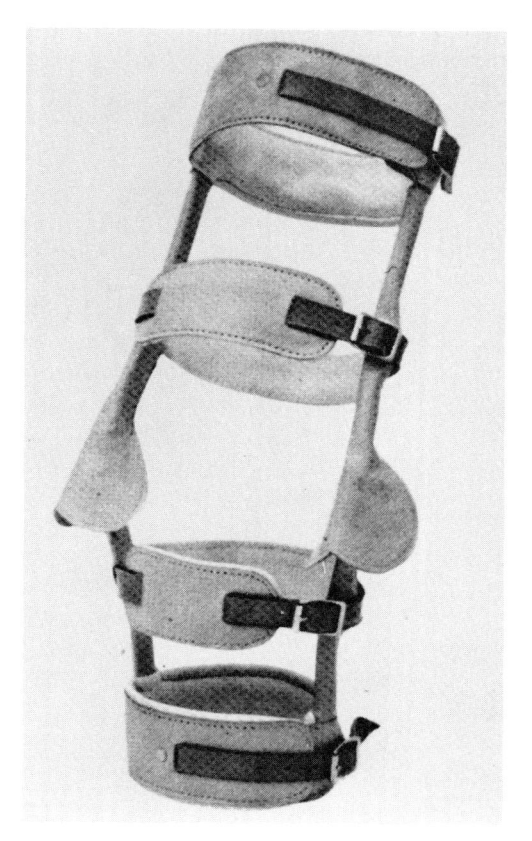

Fig. 90. Howard Marsh knee cage showing leather guards over the knee joints.

straps. At knee level is a free moving joint, allowing flexion and extension of the knee.

Measurements. The following measurements are taken:

(1) Circumference of the leg at mid-thigh level.
(2) Circumference of the leg 5 in. (13 cm) below the fibular head.
(3) The length from mid-thigh to knee joint.
(4) The length from the knee joint to 5 in. (13 cm) below the fibular head.

This splint is used when stability of the knee joint is required with movement. It also helps to prevent hyperextension of the knee and the joint then having an extension limit. It should only be used if the hip and ankle are sound.

13
Below-knee irons

Below-knee irons are used for a variety of conditions and there is a choice of design. They have the advantage of being easy to wear. All shoes have to be tubed. Footwear should ideally have a broad heel and preferably lace up with uppers that are not too shallow.

The two measurements needed for all types of irons are: (1) the length of the leg from just below the fibular head to the plantar surface of the heel; and (2) the circumference of the leg just below the fibular head. The length measurement should never be too long, as the patient will have difficulty in fully flexing the knee. Fastenings are usually Velcro or strap and buckle, and all the irons have an ankle strap to prevent the pegs from slipping out of the tubes. Childrens irons have adjustable ends for growth adjustment. The metal used is either duralamin or double sheer steel.

Double Below-Knee Iron with Round Pegs

This splint gives stability to the ankle joint, at the same time allowing movement at the ankle joint.

Double Below-Knee Iron with Flat Ends

This splint (Fig. 92) gives stability to, and prevents movement at, the ankle joint. The flat ends at the base of the irons fit into a flat socket in the heel of the shoe and prevents plantar and dorsiflexion of the ankle. Mechanically it is not a satisfactory splint, being particularly hard on the wear of the heel of the shoe. It is useful if it is necessary to rest the ankle and a walking plaster is not advisable.

Inside Iron and Outside T-Strap

The inside iron is placed down the medial side of the leg. The top is attached to a circular leather calf band just below the fibular head, and the lower end fits into the tube of the heel. The T-strap is attached to the outer side of the middle part of the shoe at the base of the upper. It is roughly triangular in shape, and ends in two straps

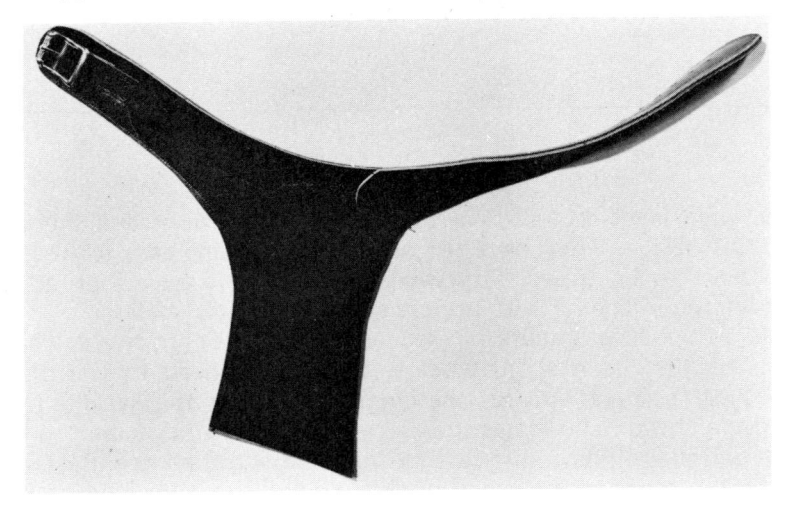

Fig. 91. A T-strap.

which fasten on the **outside** of the inside iron. The tension of the T-strap fastening on the outer side of the iron provides a corrective pull. This combination helps to correct a varus deformity of the foot, the strap always being placed on the opposite side of the deformity. Thus a relapsed club foot, one with weakness or paralysis of the peroneals, or the hemiplegic foot may benefit from this splint.

Outside Iron and Inside T-Strap

This (Fig. 92) is a more usual combination, the inside T-strap giving the corrective pull for valgus deformities of the foot. It is very often combined with a wedge heel on the inner side of the heel, $\frac{3}{16}$ in. (4·5 mm) for a child, and $\frac{1}{4}$ in. (6 mm) for the adult. The congenital condition of calcaneo valgus and the spasmodic flat foot do well with this splint. The T-strap should fit well under the arch of the foot and not be placed too far forward. It should help support the longitudinal arch and not be too big if it is to be used for the valgus foot.

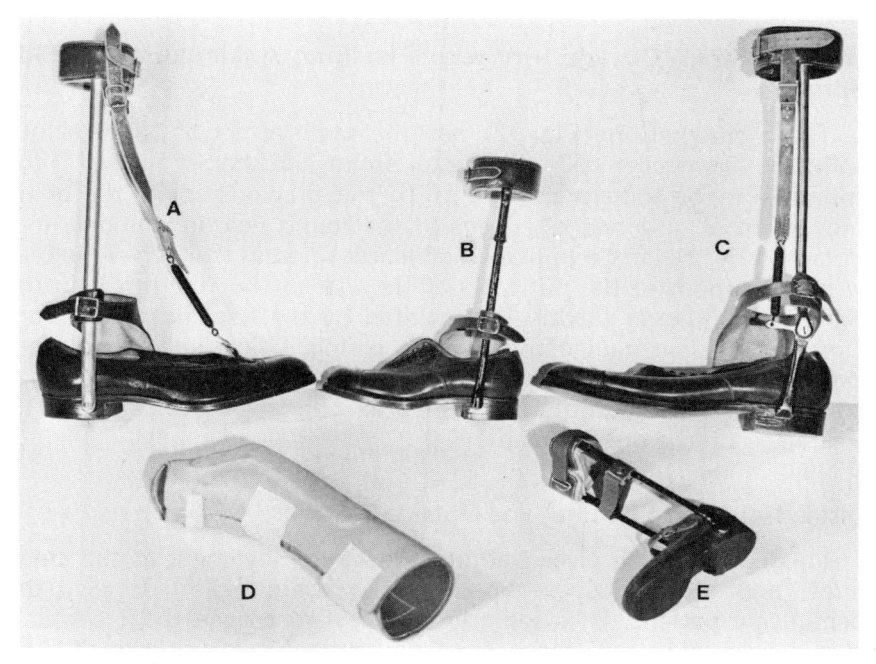

Fig. 92. (a) Inside T-strap, outside iron with centre toe-raising spring; (b) inside T-strap, outside iron; (c) inside T-strap, outside iron with flat socket ankle joint and side spring to help the dropped everted foot; (d) moulded leather anklet to give stability to the ankle joint; (e) double below knee iron to give stability to the ankle.

Outside Iron, Inside T-Strap and Centre Toe-Raising Spring

In cases of paralysis or weakness of the anterior tibial group of muscles, there is a combination of inversion and dropping of the foot. The inside T-strap helps inversion, and the toe raising spring helps to prevent plantar flexion. The spring is attached to the centre of the shoe just below the toes by means of a metal ring. The upper end of the spring is fixed to a 'Y' shaped leather strap which is fastened to the front of the calf band by adjustable straps and buckles. The tension of the spring being sufficient to prevent the toe touching the ground on walking. This is an excellent splint (Fig. 93) for the growing child or as a temporary one for the adult. It is comparatively cheap and quick to make.

Inside T-Strap, Outside Iron with Flat End, Ankle Joint and Side Spring

This combination (Fig. 92) has the same effect as the previous splint but is mechanically the better splint and should be used if the splint is to be a permanent one. In the previous splint the ankle movement is obtained by means of the round peg, in this one, it is obtained by the ankle joint being incorporated in the iron. The joint is placed opposite the patient's ankle and so the fulcrum is in the right place. Plantar flexion is prevented by the flat end of the iron. Dorsiflexion is obtained by the side spring which is attached from the ankle joint to the lower end of the iron, and the T-strap of course, inverts the foot. Note that all this structure, except the T-strap, is on the outside of the leg.

Inside Iron with Flat End, and Outside T-Strap

This combination gives stability, prevents movement at the ankle joint, and also helps eversion. It is a useful splint to give the hemiplegic patient. It is sometimes necessary to pad the T-strap. If elastic laces are used, the patient will probably be able to put the splint on unaided.

Double Below-Knee Iron with Internal Coil

This double below-knee iron has small square pegs fitting into a square socket in the shoe. This socket is attached to a wire coil which controls the plantar and dorsiflexion of the foot. It is concealed between the uppers and the soles of the shoes. The amount of dorsiflexion required depends on the angle that the peg is inserted into the shoe. This splint eliminates an obvious external toe spring.

Double Below-Knee Iron with an Exeter Coil

This splint (Fig. 93) has a coil at each lower end of the irons to prevent plantar flexion and help dorsiflexion. It needs a special tube for the shoe. It is most suitable for a small child rather than adults as it will not stand up to hard wear.

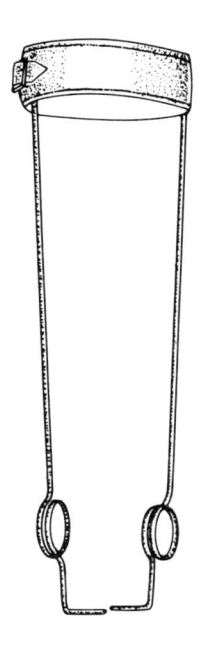

Fig. 93. Double below-knee iron with Exeter coil to prevent dropped foot.

Double Below-Knee Iron with Back Check Stops

The check stops are metal phalanges attached to a plate which is inserted above the sole of the shoe. These phalanges come just behind the lowest ends of the double iron. Each time a step is taken the iron comes into contact with the stop and so prevents plantar flexion. The metal insertion makes the shoe heavy and the constant contact between iron and stops exerts a considerable strain on the heel of the shoe and so causes necessity for repairs. A toe-raising spring is preferable if any recovery of the muscle or nerve is expected, or if the muscle is merely weak. The use of a back check stop eliminates the use of any muscle power and so is useful for the flail foot.

The Inside Iron with Flat End and Outside T-Strap

This is a very useful combination for the hemiplegic patient (Fig. 94). The flat end prevents a drop foot, and the outside T-straps help eversion. If Velcro fastenings and elastic shoe laces are used, the patient can probably manage to put the splint on unaided.

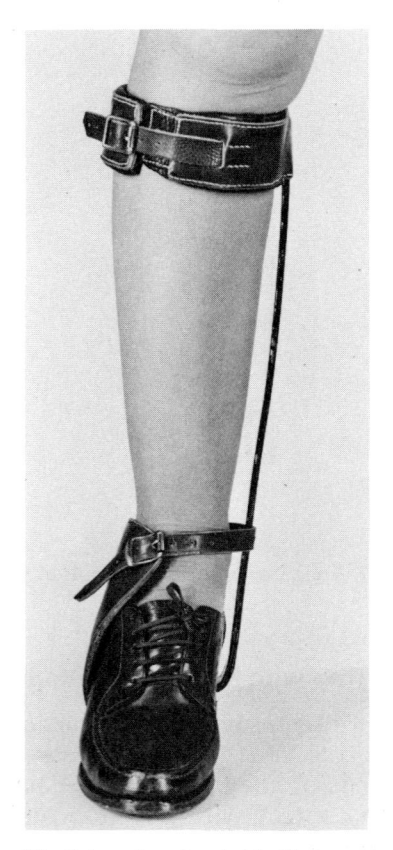

Fig. 94. Inside iron with flat end and outside T-strap, to prevent inversion and dropped foot. Useful for the hemiplegic patient.

Double Below-Knee Iron with Front Check Stop

This has the reverse action as the previous splint, the front check stop preventing dorsiflexion due to weakness or absence of the plantar flexion, usually a congenital anomaly. A combination of double below-knee irons with front and back check stops eliminates ankle movement. If the angle of the stops is widened, a little movement can be obtained if desired.

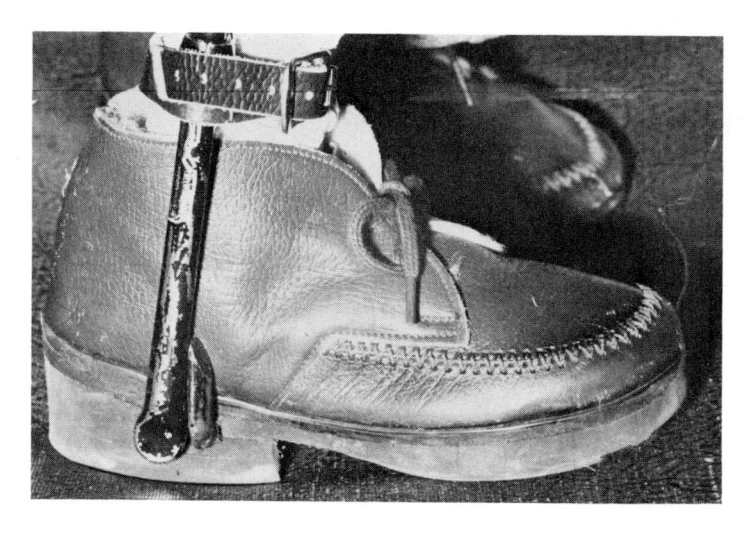

Fig. 95. Double below knee iron with front check straps for congenital deformity.

Moulded Leather Anklet

This moulded leather splint is worn next to the skin inside the shoe (Fig. 92). It is used for the flail foot in the growing child awaiting stabilization of the foot, or for the adult with disease of the bones of the foot or ankle. Difficulty may be had in getting the foot and splint into the shoe. It is advisable to use a lace-up shoe which can have the opening split down to the toes and a long lace for fastening the shoe. The foot within the splint can then be laid into the shoe.

Measurements are taken by means of a plaster cast from the base of the toes to about 5 in. above the ankle. This splint can also be made in polythene, although it is less pliable and very much more difficult to apply.

Yates Splint for Dropped Foot

This splint has a good cosmetic appearance, and is worn next to the skin beneath the stocking. It is a polythene back splint just covering the sole of the foot and back of the leg with a Velcro fastening at the top. This prevents the foot from dropping and makes the gait natural.

The Shoe Clasp Ankle-Foot Orthosis

This posterior orthosis is designed to prevent drop foot in the patient with a mild valgus or varus deformity. Its great advantages are that it is not noticeable and can be interchanged with other shoes.

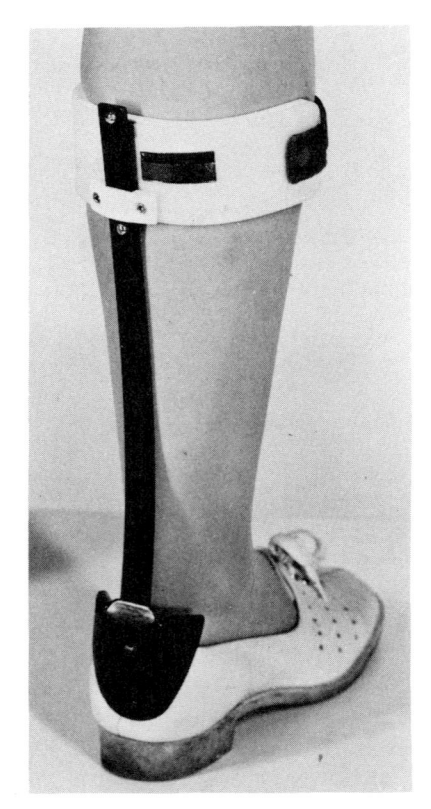

Fig. 96. Shoe clasp with dropped foot splint.

The shoes, however, should be of the lace-up, broad-heeled variety. The counter of the shoe should be strong. The calf rod and calf hand are polypropylene. Both are flexible enough to accommodate the shape of the leg. The lower end of the posterior rod is attached to a clasp. This clasp grips the back of the shoe and should end $\frac{1}{8}$ in. (3 mm) above the sole of the shoe. The clasp can be adjusted by a pair of pliers to fit the shoe closely, especial care being taken on the inner side, it should lie flat against the counter and avoid infringement on the Achilles tendon. The upper edge of the calf band should lie at the level of the maximum diameter of the calf. The posterior bar can be cut off after measurement and attached to the calf band by two screws. If a strong dorsiflexion is required, the top edge of the clasp which connects with the bar, can be bent forward towards the bar. This will tilt the bar forwards, thus increasing resistance to plantar flexion. Velcro fastening is used for the calf band. The calf band does not, as a rule, have to be padded but $\frac{3}{16}$ in. (4·5 mm) foam can be used, if needed. This apparatus is supplied in a standard size which can be altered as required.

14
Congenital foot deformity splints

CLUB FOOT SPLINTS

The congenital deformity of the club foot baby is one of equinovarus, therefore splintage is designed to give over correction in the calcaneovalgus position of the foot.

Strapping Correction

The condition is usually diagnosed soon after the birth of the baby. If the condition is mild, or if a splint is not immediately available strapping can be applied.

Application. The knee is held at right angles, a roll of 1 in. strapping is passed over the flexed knee and round the forefoot maintaining dorsiflexion and eversion of the foot. In some cases two strips of strapping may be necessary. Some circular strips of strapping may also be necessary to keep the longer strips in place. The skin should be treated first with Tinc Benzco. The strapping should be applied for not longer than 1 week and should be removed with the help of 'Zoff', the skin is then cleaned, manipulation is carried out and then either re-application of the strapping or splint.

Denis Browne Splint for Club Feet

The Denis Browne splint (Figs 97 and 98) maintains a correction but does not correct the deformity, thus it should be possible to

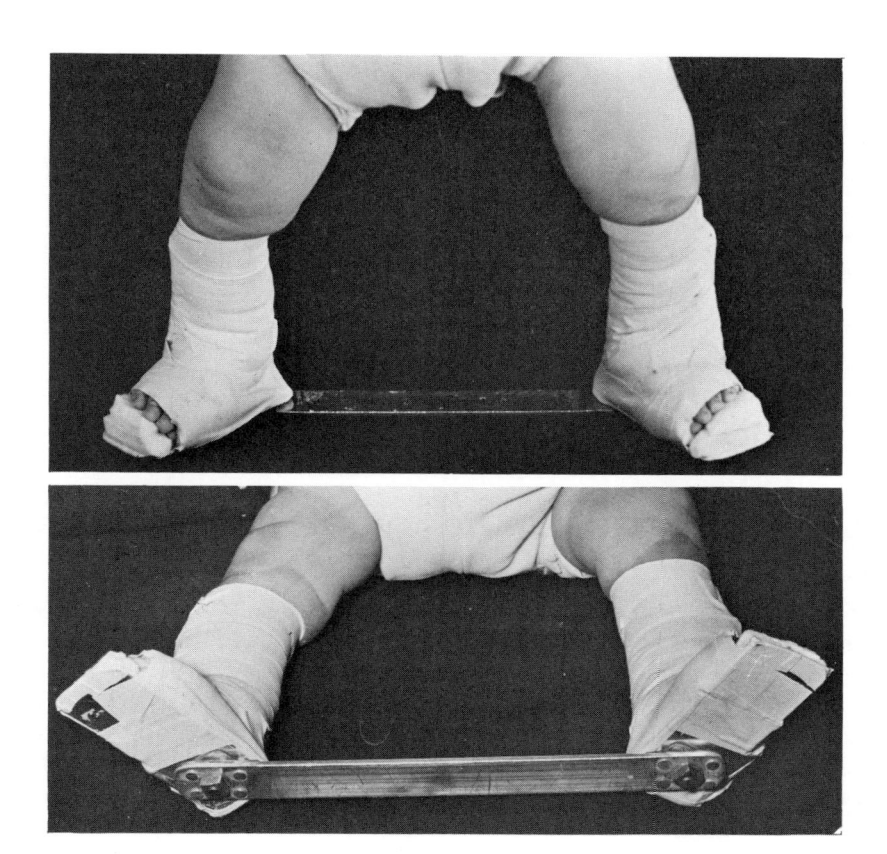

Fig. 97. The Denis Browne splint applied. (Top) Note eversion of foot pieces and position of the eversion pads. (Bottom) Showing under surface.

passively correct the deformity before the splint is applied. If little or no correction can be obtained by manipulation, then serial plasters should be applied until over correction can be obtained. The feet are then ready for the application of Denis Browne splints. The splints are usually worn for 9 months to 1 year, until the child can stand, and are made in a succession of sizes. They consist of a pair of metal foot splints joined by a cross bar. The foot splints are made up of a rectangular foot plate with a lateral leg plate continuing from the posterior outer edge of the foot plate. The leg plates which extend to above the external malleolic are covered with adhesive felt. The foot plates have serrated discs permanently riveted to the back of the

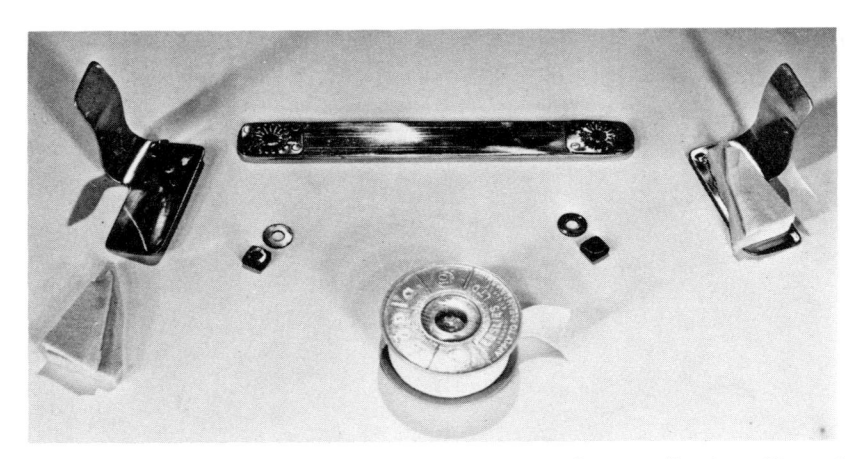

Fig. 98. The Denis Browne club foot splint before application. Note the triangular felt pads to give eversion of the foot.

under surface, through which bolts are pressed. Matching serrated discs are riveted to each end of the cross bar. A wing nut is used to fix the foot plate in position.

The correction of the foot into calcaneovalgus is carried out by two graded triangular adhesive felt pads which are placed on the foot plates. An understanding of the correction desired is necessary for correct positioning of the pads. The pads are placed in such a way that the greatest depth is on the front and outer sides of the foot plates, so that the heels and inner borders of the feet are placed straight on to the foot plates—the area of the plates not covered by the triangular pads are covered with either strapping or thin adhesive felt.

Application. The baby's skin should be cleaned with 'Zoff' and covered with Tinc Benzco. The splint should be covered with felt and strapping. The forefoot should be fixed first with two rounds of 1-in. (2·5-cm) strapping, the heel is next strapped to the splint, and lastly the leg plate is strapped to the baby's leg. If the foot is properly strapped in the plantar grade position when the leg plate is brought into contact with the leg, a few degrees of eversion is obtained. The bar is next screwed to the foot plates, with the feet in 60 degrees of eversion. The eversion can be increased at each application. The baby helps with the correction by constant kicking, which at the same time strengthens the leg muscles. This splint, ideally, should be changed at weekly intervals, the skin inspected, the feet manipulated, and active eversion encouraged. When the splint is left off the baby wears a splint at night and has outside sole and heel wedges of $\frac{3}{16}$ in. (4·5 mm) applied to little lace up shoes. The outside wedges maintaining the eversion of the foot.

Hobble Night Splint

This splint (Fig. 99) is worn at night when the baby is released from the Denis Browne splint or plasters. It is a soft leather boot with metal sole plate, a calf band and mid-thigh bands. The calf band is joined to the top of the boot by two adjustable bars. The boot is open at the toe. The sole plate has an adjustable extended $\frac{1}{2}$-in. (12-mm) bar which lies laterally to the boot. The end of the bar has a socket through which the corrective leather strap passes, which in turn is fixed to the outer side of the calf band. This strap maintains dorsiflexion and eversion. The knee is flexed and kept in position by the thigh cuff and so prevents the foot from being pulled out of the boot. The calf bars can be elongated as the child grows, and the toes can protrude through the boot. It should be remembered that the baby may resent being so restricted, and that the mother should fully understand how to apply the splint. The boot is laced and sometimes an interior strap is fixed over the front of the ankle to keep the heel down. This splint may be worn for 1 to 3 years, or until the child becomes stronger than the splint. The alternative is a plaster night splint or the Robert Jones club foot shoe.

Measurements. The following measurements are taken:
 (1) Circumference of the mid-thigh.
 (2) Circumference of the leg at the level of the fibular head.
 (3) Circumference of the leg just above the ankle.
 (4) Circumference of the heel and front of the ankle.
 (5) Circumference of the instep.
 (6) Length from mid-thigh to the back of the knee joint (with knee flexed).
 (7) Length from the back of the knee joint to the plantar surface of the heel.
 (8) Length from the back of the heel to the tip of the hallux.

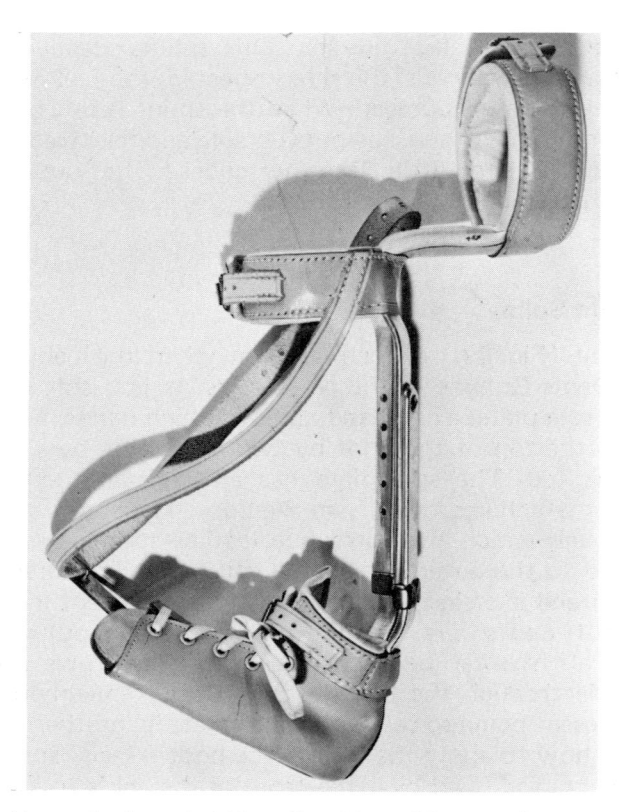

Fig. 99. Above the knee hobble splint. Note the corrective strap to maintain dorsiflexion and eversion.

This splint may be used bilaterally as below knee splints and fixed to a hinged bar. The bar joins both feet and is hinged at either end, which allows free ankle movement.

Robert Jones Club Foot Shoe

This splint consists of a padded aluminium trough which extends from below the fibular head to above the ankle. It is connected to a padded foot plate which has side flanges, by a malleable bar or ball and socket type joint (Fig. 100). Thus the corrective position of dorsiflexion and eversion can be adjusted and fixed. The necessary retaining straps fix the leg and foot. Note that the heel is left free.

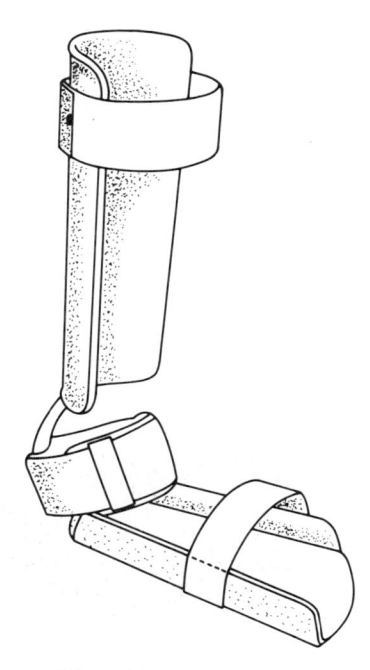

Fig. 100. Club foot shoe.

Boots on a Bar

A simple boot modification can be used as a night splint. A pair of well fitting boots can be fixed to a bar (Fig. 101). The boot should be in at least 60 degrees of eversion. The conditions of metatarsus varus and persistent fetal alignment can use this splint. The width of the bars vary with the size of the child but starts at 8 in. (20 cm). The shoes are reversed if the condition being treated is a metatarsus varus.

FOOT SPLINTS

Banana Splint

This splint (Fig. 102) is used for correcting the congenital deformity of calcaneovalgus. It is a banana shaped piece of metal, which should be covered on the slightly concave side with adhesive felt. It is usually made in a series of graded lengths from 4 to 7 in. (10 to 18 cm), and all lengths are approximately 1 in. (2·5 cm) wide.

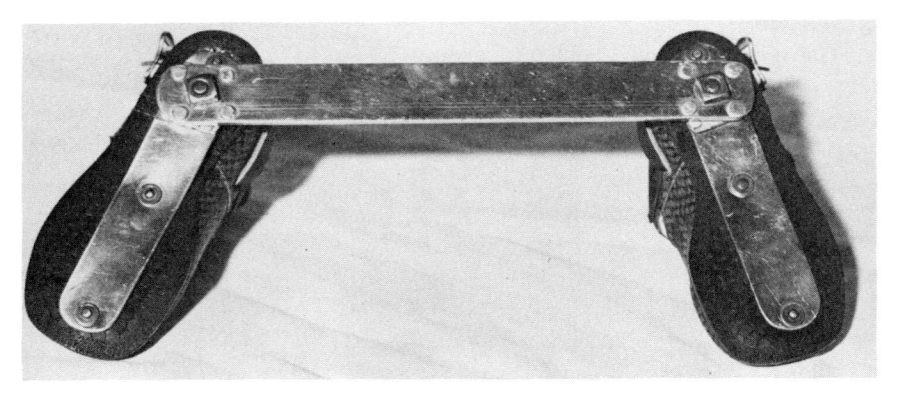

Fig. 101. Boots on a bar.

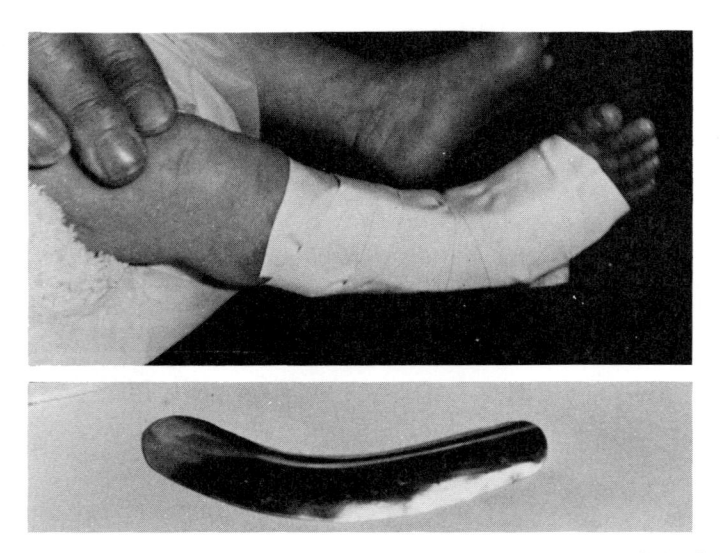

Fig. 102. Baby with banana splint strapped to the outer side of the foot and ankle.

Application. The splint is applied as soon as possible after birth. The foot is held in the equinovarus position, the splint being placed on the outer side of the foot and leg. The skin should first be covered with Tinc Benzco, and the splint is fixed with 1 in. (2·5 cm) strapping. The toes should be left free, and the circulation watched. The splint is changed at weekly intervals, a period of 3 to 4 weeks being sufficient. The mother continues the treatment with passive manipulations in the over-corrected position.

The Bristol Combined Strapping and Sole Plate for Club Feet Correction

The combination of club feet strapping incorporating a sole plate can be used to correct the equinovarus deformity of club feet (Fig. 103). The metal sole plate which should extend from the back of the heel to about ½ in. (12 mm) beyond the toes is covered with adhesive felt or sorbo. One-inch strapping is used to maintain the correction.

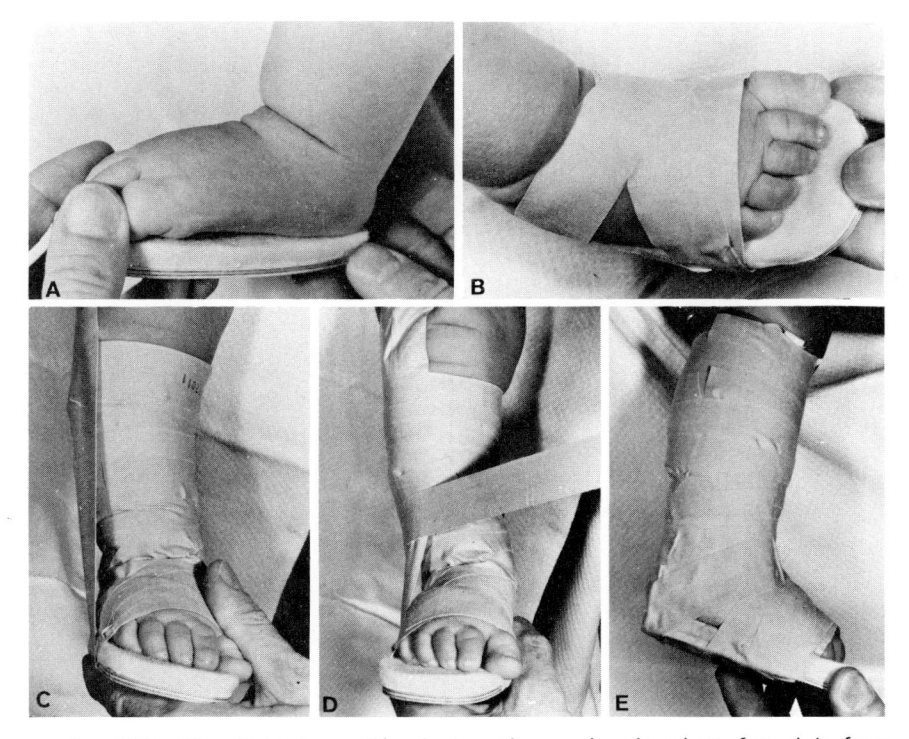

Fig. 103. The Bristol combined strapping and sole plate for club foot correction: (a) babies foot placed on metal foot piece; (b) first turns of strapping applied; (c) strapping applied to full length of lower leg with the addition of the eversion length of strapping; (d) the eversion length of strapping being overstrapped; (e) strapping completed.

Method. The foot should be held plantar-grade on the sole plate. The strapping is then applied twice round the forefoot and finishes round the back of the heel and across the under surface of the forefoot where it is cut. Eversion strapping is then applied from the toes to just below the knee, nicking it in places so that it accommodates the calf comfortably. Two lengths of strapping are next applied under the forefront of the foot and up the outer side of the leg. These strips should be fixed tightly so that the whole foot is brought into eversion. Finally more strapping is applied from the knee to the toes, without in, to keep the two lengths in position and so maintain evasion. This form of splinting is changed at weekly or fortnightly intervals and the skin cleaned in the usual way with 'Zoff' or ether meth. Tinc Benzco can be used to protect the skin before application of the strapping.

15
Insoles and shoe adaptations

Insoles are a simple way of helping the weak and painful foot without the shoe having to be adapted. It is however, sometimes necessary to wear a half size larger shoe than normal. It is always best to wear a broad heeled shoe and preferably a lace-up one.

Domed Insole

This is a leather insole (Fig. 104) with the addition of a metatarsal dome. The dome is a firm triangular pad incorporated into the insole and is usually fixed between an upper thin leather covering and the firm sole itself. The position is important, it should be *behind* the metatarsal heads. If it was under the metatarsal heads it would increase the pressure in the painful area. Some of the body weight is taken off the metatarsal heads if it is correctly placed, and the toes should fall into a straighter position. The measurements are taken by either a tracing of the foot, or, if the foot is normal in shape it is only necessary to take the size of the shoe. It may be easier when fitting a female shoe to have the insole made a half size smaller than the shoe size. In any case it is most satisfactory when fitting the insole to trim it to fit the shoe, taking care that the dome is in the correct place.

Rose's Insole

This is an insole (Fig. 104) which is a graded metatarsal bar ending in a roll which again fits behind the metatarsal heads, so that the medial edge is further forward than the lateral edge.

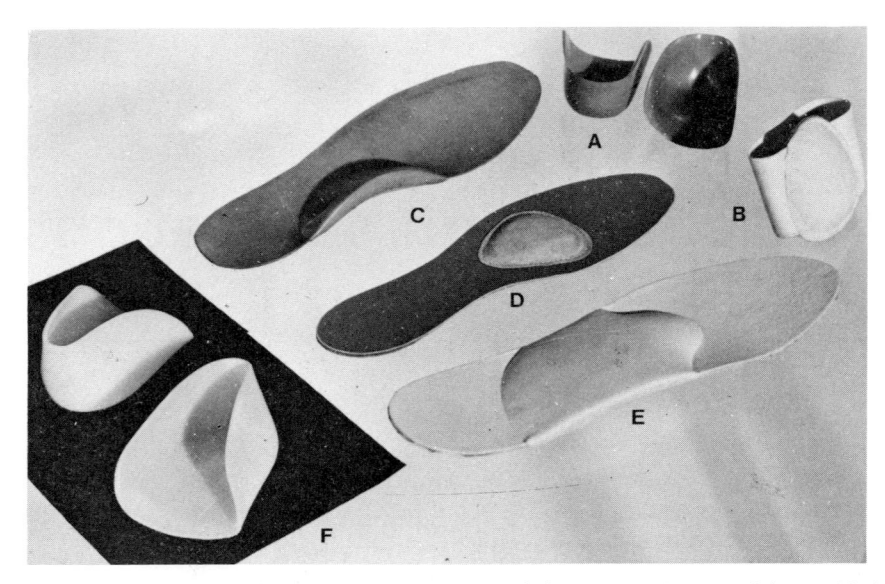

Fig. 104. (a) and (f) Polythene heel caps; (b) metatarsal strap; (c) moulded leather arch support; (d) domed insole; (e) Rose's insole.

Moulded Leather Arch Support

The moulded leather arch support (Fig. 104) or insole with the valgus lift, takes up a certain amount of room in the shoe, is again best in a shoe larger than the normal size. The lift is made of firm sponge rubber which is covered with leather, and it lies under the longitudinal arch. The measurements are as for domed insoles, but if a tracing of the outline is taken, the area of the longitudinal arch can be marked as well.

Domed Arch Support

This is a combination of the domed insole and moulded leather arch support.

Soft Insole

Some patients suffer from tender feet with callosities. A plain sorbo rubber insole often helps, with excavations cut where callouses give trouble.

Plastazote Insoles

These are very helpful as they are so resilient though their life is short and the patient should have two pairs made. The Plastazote is heated and placed on a thick pad of felt or 1-in. (2·5-cm) Plastazote. The patient stands with full weight on the feet and the Plastazote is moulded to the patient's feet whilst it cools. It needs careful trimming to enable it to fit well into the patient's shoe.

Whitman's Sole Plate

The Whitman's sole plate (Fig. 105) is a rigid duralumin support with an arch support and outer lip to help keep the foot compressed. It has a sharp peg at it's posterior under surface to fix it to the shoe. It is used for the elderly patient with an osteo-arthritic foot, the patient with a rigid painful flat foot, and the patient with an osteomyelitis of the tarsus after plaster fixation. The measurements are taken by a plaster cast of the foot with the arches well moulded. The splint relieves the foot of some of the body weight and once they are worn, the patient finds it difficult to give them up. The metal is usually covered with leather as it can corrode with the heat of the foot. Alternatively, polythene, Darvic or Prenyl supports can be worn.

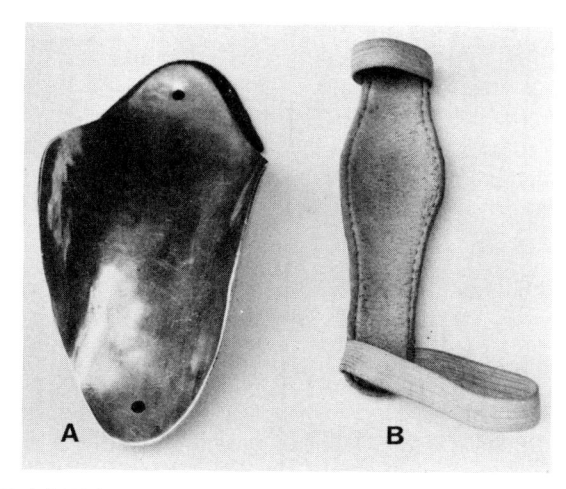

Fig. 105. (a) Whitman's sole plate, and (b) hallux valgus night splint.

Metal Arch Supports

The Dr Scholl's type of metal arch support is similar to the Whitman's sole plate, but it does not have the outer lip.

Metatarsal Strap

This is an elastic garter with a leather covered pad attached to it. It is worn round the forefoot, the pad lying behind the metatarsal heads. It is often used after surgery of the hallux and helps to compress the foot. The measurement is the circumference of the forefoot.

Hallux Valgus Night Splint

This is a useful night splint for the patient with the incipient hallux valgus. The big toe should not be rigid and the patient should be able to exercise the abductor hallucis muscle.

Heel Cap

Heel caps are worn next to the skin inside the shoes. They enclose the heels and extend forwards to the navicular. They hold the heel in the neutral position, thus correcting a valgus or varus heel. The material used can be polythene, Prenyl or Polypropylane. Stock sizes may be kept, but if they are being worn for the valgus foot, plaster casts may be taken. The longitudinal arch should be well moulded and the heel held quite straight, and the foot at a right angle. They are comfortable and effective to wear. It is preferable for the shoes to have broad heels and laces.

TOE SPLINTS

Halux Valgus Night Splint

The splint is a thin leather covered duralumin splint which lies down the inside of the foot. It has elastic fastenings which encircle the instep and big toe and so keeps the toe straight. It should only be worn at night.

Measurements. The following measurements are taken:
   (1) Length from the top of the hallux to the navicular.
   (2) The circumference of the instep.
   (3) The circumference of the hallux.

Metal Toe Splints

There are a variety of toe splints which can be worn after surgery. They are usually made in a range of sizes. In shape they are a narrow $\frac{1}{2}$-in. (1·2-cm) plate ending in a round broader section. The narrow end is placed under the distal end of the toe. The splints are usually covered with strapping or adhesive felt, and are kept in position by a narrow bandage or $\frac{1}{2}$-in. (1·2-cm) strapping.

SHOE ALTERATIONS

Toe Blocks for Use in Amputation of Toes

Patients who have had all their toes amputated have difficulty with their footwear. Lace-up shoes should be worn, and unless the space left by the absence of the toes is filled up the shoes will buckle at the distal end of the foot and will appear unnatural. Insoles with cork blocks can be inserted in the shoes. A tracing of the foot should be taken. This tracing with the required shoe enables the cork insert to be made to fit the shoe. The cork block is covered with leather and forms part of the insole and can thus be used for more than one pair of shoes.

The Oswestry Moccasin

This useful moccasin (Fig. 106) is used for the patient with one foot larger than the other. It allows the patient to wear shoes of equal sizes in spite of a severe foot discrepancy. A moccasion of basil leather is made to the size of the larger foot. The intervening gap between the edge of the moccasin and the toes is filled with Plastazote. The appliance is worn under the stocking, thus enabling shoes of equal size to be worn.

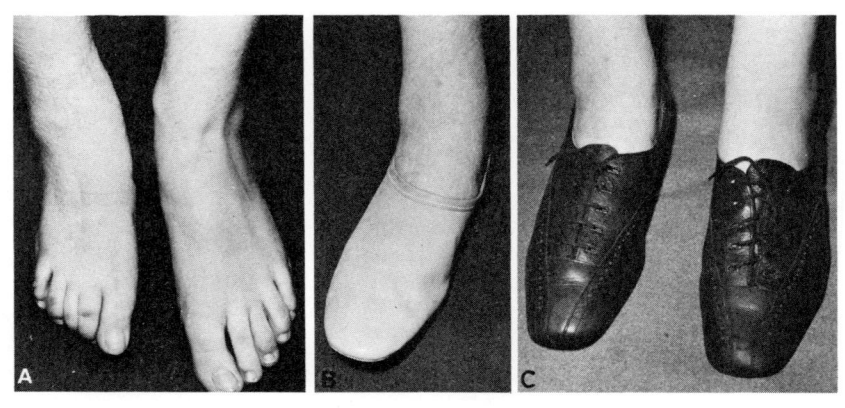

Fig. 106. (a) Patient with foot discrepancy, (b) the Oswestry moccasin, (c) the finished shoes.

Inside Heel Wedge

This is the simplest and commonest shoe alteration and is used for postural flat feet and knock knees (Fig. 107). Ideally a leather heel is most suitable. The heel is removed, a taper wedge inserted at the top, with the deepest part of the wedge on the inner side, and the heel re-applied. Shoes with composition heels or welded footwear have to have the wedge stuck at the base of the heel, so it is the first part to be worn, whereas if inserted at the top of the heel, it is there for the life of the shoe. Childrens shoes have a $\frac{3}{16}$-in. (4·5-mm) inside wedge, large children and adults a $\frac{1}{4}$-in. (6-mm) inner wedge, and in extreme cases a $\frac{3}{8}$-in. (9-mm) inner wedge can be used.

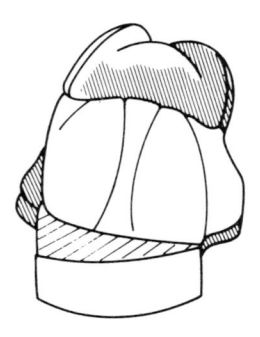

Fig. 107. Shoe showing inside wedge heel.

Outside Wedges

Children with treated talipes equinovarus can wear a $\frac{3}{16}$-in. (4·5-mm) outside wedge to sole and heel.

Inside Heel Wedge, Outside Sole Wedge

This combination is used for small children who turn their toes in, or who wear their shoes out excessively with just an inner wedge.

Thomas or Extended Heel

In cases of severe flat feet it may be necessary to extend the depth of the heel on the inner side beyond the arch of the foot. This is combined with an inner wedge.

Inside or Outside Floats of Flares

The base of the heel may be broadened on the inner or outer sides, or both sides of the heel. This is a very simple and effective remedy for the patient who has a strained or sprained internal or external colateral ligaments of the ankle joints. It is very difficult to turn the ankle on the side of the extended width of the heel. The outer flare of the heel can be used in conjunction with an inner wedge of the heel. Sometimes the child with a wedge heel on the inner side wears the uppers over on the outer side—an outside flare will prevent this.

Hallux Rigidus Crook

This is a $\frac{1}{4}$-in. (6-mm) layer of leather, tapered to the outer side, which is fixed to the sole underneath the hallux. It has the effect of tipping some of the body weight away from the big toe, at the same time stiffening the area beneath the big toe—this is a stiff and painful condition. It can also be combined with a metatarsal roll.

Varus Plate

In cases of metatarsus varus when the forefoot is mobile, the inner border of the foot can be kept straight by the insertion of a $\frac{1}{2}$-in. (12-mm) thin duralumin plate. This is placed between the outer leather and the lining and extends from the top of the hallux to the beginning of the instep. Reverse shoes can also be worn for this condition.

Metatarsal Bar

This simple remedy is a $\frac{1}{4}$-in. (6-mm) thick strip of leather, $\frac{1}{2}$-in. (12-mm) wide, placed on the sole behind the metatarsal heads (Fig. 108). This takes some of the body weight off the metatarsal heads.

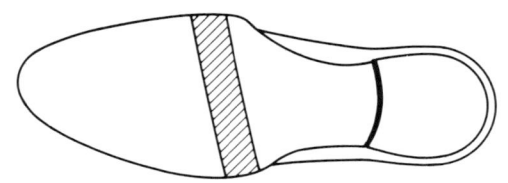

Fig. 108. Shoe showing metatarsal bar. Note that the bar is well behind the metatarsal heads.

Metatarsal Rocker Bars

This is a similarly placed bar to the metatarsal bar but more refined in that it is rounded in shape.

Shoe Raises

The type of raise is dependent on the length of time it has to be worn, the type of shoe to be raised, and the amount of raise required.

Temporary Raise

This is used when a raise is required to equalize the length of the legs when either a walking plaster is being worn on one leg, or an appliance which keeps the knee straight. It may also be worn when crutches are used and non-weight bearing of one leg is required. One inch or more can be fixed to the heel and sole of the good foot. A temporary raise may be used for the patient who has had a pseudarthrosis of the hip, when the shortening varies for a time. A temporary raise is more easily altered. When the hip has become stable, and the shortening unvaried, a cork raise can be inserted.

Temporary raises are usually wood covered with leather or the same composition as the original shoe's sole and heel. Uncovered cork can also be used as well as layers of leather. The raises are usually stuck on to the shoe, or in the case of wooden blocks, nailed. In any case it should be possible to remove the raise with a lever when it is no longer required.

Cork or Permanent Raise

Cork is the lightest substance to use as a raise, which gives additional weight to be borne. It should be carried out by surgical boot makers, as a certain amount of skill is required, the tapering varies according to the pitch of the shoe. The cork is inserted between the uppers and sole and heel, and covered with leather to match the shoe (Fig. 109). The patient's own shoes can be raised. If, however, a surgical shoe is being made the cork is included in the uppers, these being deep enough to include the cork. A 'through raise' is one which does not vary in depth, it usually ends an inch or two short of the toes, to make walking easier. A tapered raise is one which is decreased in depth from the sole towards the toes. A 1-in.

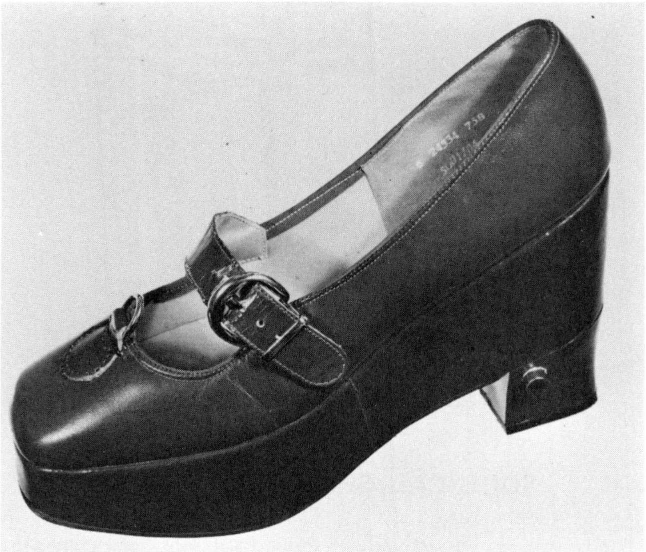

Fig. 109. Shoe with cork raise inserted above the caliper tube.

(2·5-cm) tapered raise would probably be ½-in. (12-mm) sole and ¼-in. (6-mm) toe. This allows a more natural gait.

A caliper tube is often incorporated in the heel below the cork raise. It should be remembered when measuring a patient who has a leg shortening for a caliper that the amount of shortening should be added to the length of the caliper, as the tube is at the base of the raise. If the length is omitted, when the caliper is tried on, it will be too short, being minus the required raise. A temporary raise is always fixed to the shoe below the caliper tube. If the amount of shortening is 4 in. (10 cm) or more, the patient may prefer to wear a pattern (Fig. 110). This is metal framework designed to fit the base of the shoe. It is extremely unsightly, but some patients find it easier to manage than a deep cork raise.

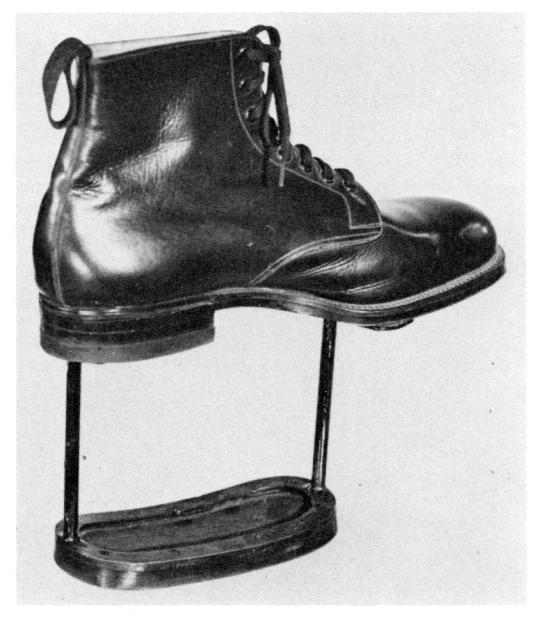

Fig. 110. Shoe showing a 5-in. (13-cm) patten.

SURGICAL SHOES OR BOOTS

Surgical footwear is used when the feet are abnormally shaped, where there is excessive shorterning of the leg whether due to polio in childhood or hip disease, or in untreated congenital abnormalities. The function of the footwear is to distribute the weight which has to be carried by the deformed foot, so as to avoid excessive pressure on any one point. Therefore the shoe must really fit the foot, with the use of built-in insoles or supports to relieve pressure on prominent bony points. If there are displaced or claw toes, soft uppers should be used. If the foot is rigid or flail, the shoe should be opened to the toes and long laces used; it is otherwise extremely difficult to get the shoes on. It is not usually satisfactory to attempt to correct the foot. The cosmetic appearance of the surgical shoe often leaves a lot to be desired, but comfort and function are more important. Felt uppers may be used where softness and lightness are essential. Cork inserts vary very much in shape according to the deformity present. The cork often compensates for the deformity.

Cradle Cork

This is a wide boat-shaped cork often used for the flail foot with no apparent heel.

Cork for the Untreated Talipes Equinovarus

The patient, without footwear, walks on his toes. The cork is designed to take the weight more evenly, that is, under the instep and heel, so that the depth at the heel may be as much as 5 in. (13 cm) with 1 in. (2·5 cm) at the toe.

O'Connor Extension and Cork Raise

The patient wears his own shoe within a surgical boot (Fig. 111). The cork compensator is high at the heel and slopes straight down on to the toe, the patient's own shoe resting on the cork, which helps to distribute the weight. The surgical boot unlaces to the toe and is not very sightly.

Measurements. In cases of severe deformity it is always best to take a plaster cast of the foot. When a cast is not necessary, a tracing or outline of the foot is taken. The patient should sit so that the weight of the lower leg is on the foot, and the foot is plantar-grade. The outline should be taken with either a pencil block, or the pencil held

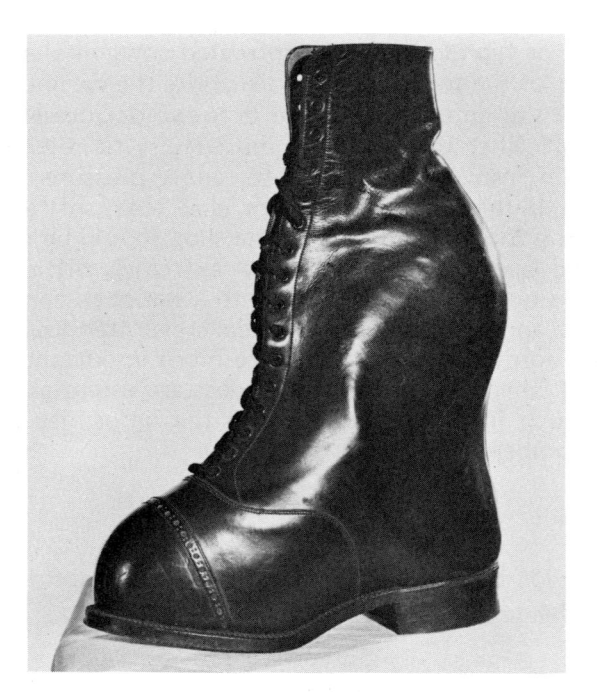

Fig. 111. O'Connor type extension boot to be worn in conjunction with normal footwear.

quite straight. With the foot still in position the following measurements should be taken:

(1) Circumference of the forefoot.
(2) Circumference of the instep.
(3) Circumference of the heel–ankle, the tape measure encircling the point of the heel and front of the ankle.

The depth of the toes should be measured, this is particularly important in patients with over-riding or claw toes, bunions should be marked on the tracings as also the position of metatarsal domes or valgus supports. This is done by slipping a finger under the desired spot by way of the instep, and marking it when the foot is raised. All surgical footwear, when being fitted for the first time, should be fitted in 'the rough'. A temporary heel and laces will be used. It is much easier to alter a shoe before the permanent soles and heels are fixed.

Providing the workshops or surgical footwear firms keep the lasts, successive pairs may be supplied without the intervening rough fitting.

Plastazote Shoes and Sandals

These are used for their extreme lightness and resiliency.

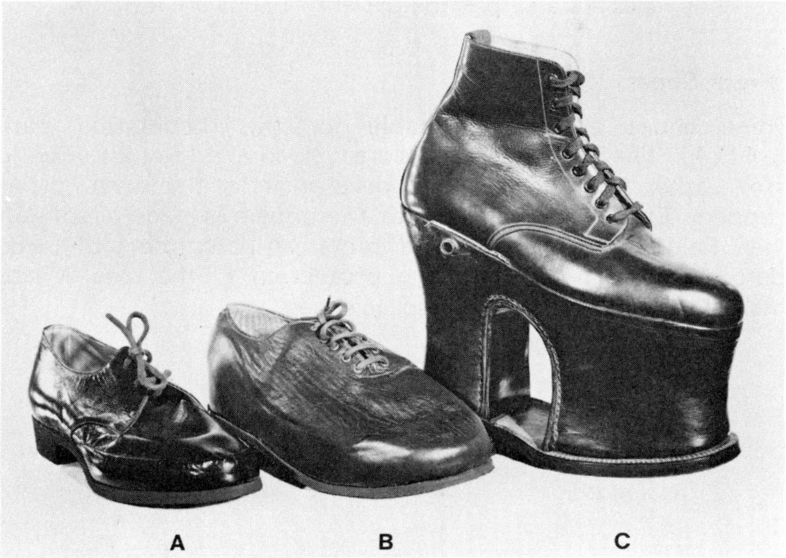

Fig. 112. (a) Ski-front surgical shoe. (b) Space shoe. (c) Shoe with deep cork raises, sometimes known as bridge cork.

Space Shoes

Space shoes (Fig. 112B) are similar in construction to the American contoured shoes. They are surgical shoes but are made without a last. The soles and heels are welded to the uppers. The uppers are made of soft glacé leather. The shoes are comfortable and suitable for the rheumatoid patient, light in weight, but unsightly to look at.

Measurements. Plaster casts of the feet should be taken, but additional measurements are not necessary. The patient should be sitting with the feet resting on the floor. A ½-in. (12-cm) block should be at hand. The patient's feet can be oiled or covered with stockinette. Plaster is applied over a centrally placed length of wire. When the plaster is setting, the ½-in. (1·2-cm) block should be placed under the heels and the patient encouraged to stand and bear weight until the plaster has set. The negative is removed in the usual manner, and the filled cast is sent to the boot shop. The front of the cast is built up by the boot maker, and the heels are shaped if necessary. Elastic shoe laces are a help if the patient's hands are affected.

Ski Front Shoes

These shoes are also suitable for the rheumatoid patient (Fig. 112A). The soles and uppers are welded and they are very light. A firm leather ring 1-in. (2·5-cm) deep encircles the lower border of the uppers. The intervening part of the uppers is made of soft single leather. Painful or overriding toe joints can be comfortably accommodated, the firm border giving protection to the toes. Measurements are the same as those for space shoes.

16
Spinal braces

Spinal braces are used to immobilize or restrict trunk movements, or to give support to the trunk.

Moulded Leather Jacket

This is a very comfortable support and is often used for the patient who needs a permanent brace (Fig. 113). Patients with an ideopathic scoliosis, tubercular spine, or polyomyelitis, come into this category. Measurements are taken by means of a plaster cast of the whole trunk, care being taken to mark areas of the skin where there are prominent bony joints with an indelible pencil. These may be the anterior superior iliac spines, a kyphos or rib bulge. It may be necessary to suspend the patient during the casting, to obtain as straight a spine as possible. The cast wire is usually placed down the centre front of the trunk, and the plaster is applied over one layer of stockinette. As in all moulded leather supports, the jacket is tried on 'in the rough' and any alterations to be made are noted. It is easy at this stage to cut away surplus leather and to have parts re-moulded. The finished product is reinforced with duralumin struts and Velcro fastenings. It is lined with chamois leather, and the outside is polished. If a jacket is being made for a patient with a kyphoscoliosis, support is given below the maximum convexity of the curve, it may be higher on the concave side. It is never desirable to bring any type of support above the maximum convexity of a curve. The top edge of the concave side often has a leather covered sorbo rubber roll for added comfort.

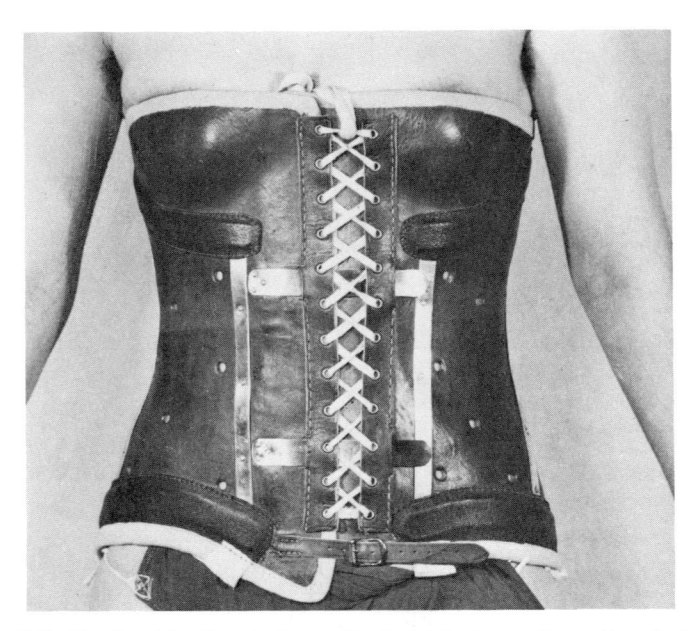

Fig. 113. Moulded leather jacket with front lacing. Alternative fastenings of Velcro or straps and buckles may be used.

Polythene Jacket

This is an alternative material, but due to its non-absorbent qualities, is not generally so comfortable. The edges too, tend to be harder. The polythene should be perforated and may be lined with sponge rubber. Some patients like to have both a leather and polythene jacket to wear on different occasions. A plaster cast is needed.

Plastazote Jacket

This is an excellent temporary jacket and is usually strengthened with polythene strips. The advantage is that it can be made straight away on the patient.

Goldthwaite Brace

One alternative to a plaster jacket is the Goldthwaite brace. It is a skeletal type of brace, the metal strips being padded and covered with leather. It is suitable for stout patients, and is more comfortable for men than women. The upper bars should lie above the nipple line and the lower bars encircle the pelvis. A plaster cast is necessary.

McKee Brace

This brace (Fig. 114) is an alternative to the Goldthwait brace. It is skeletal, with a 4 in. (10 cm) wide lumbar pad which extends the depth of the back. The front has parallel longitudinal bars with a 2 to 3 in. (5 to 7·5 cm) gap between them, over which there are three Velcro fastenings. A plaster cast of the trunk is required. It is sometimes difficult to fit, due to the rigidity of the anterior longitudinal bars. It is effective in supporting the lumbar spine and preventing flexion.

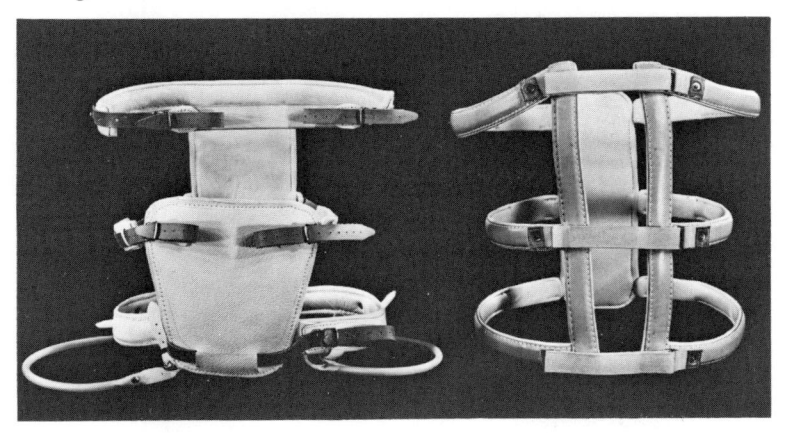

Fig. 114. A McKee brace (left) and a Goldthwaite brace (right).

Fisher Brace

This is another type of skeletal brace, which usually has axillary holds and corset front. As with other braces a plaster cast of the trunk is necessary.

Jewett Brace

The Jewett or hyperextension brace (Fig. 115) is again a metal skeletal type with three pads as corrective pressure points. The metal framework extends down on either side of the trunk, and across the upper front of the trunk and lower part of the pelvis. The upper pads lie on a level with the sternal notch and the lower pad just above the pubis. The third rectangular pad fits into the lumbar lordosis and is

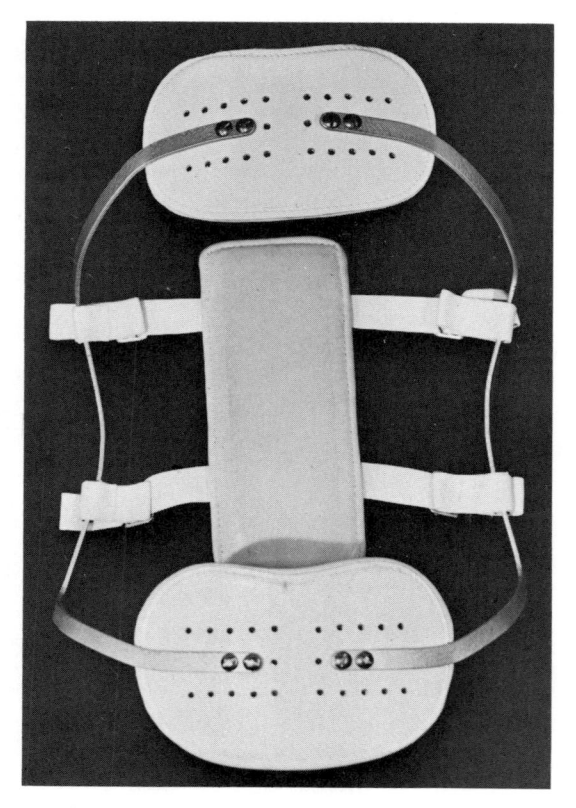

Fig. 115. Anterior view of a Jewett brace.

joined to the side struts with canvas straps. The sides of the framework are adjustable, and can be lengthened to obtain more extension of the spine. It will be seen that there is a minimum of splinting to obtain extension of the spine, the limits top and bottom anteriorly preventing flexion of the spine. The measurements are best taken by a plaster cast of the trunk.

Jones Brace

This brace has been much modified since it was first introduced in the early 1920s by Sir Robert Jones for the treatment of tuberculosis of the spine. It consists posteriorly of two parallel bars joined at the bottom by a wider horizontal bar. The two bars are joined at the top by a shallow flat hoop. The metal is usually aluminium, which is light and strong (Fig. 116). All the metal work is covered with padded

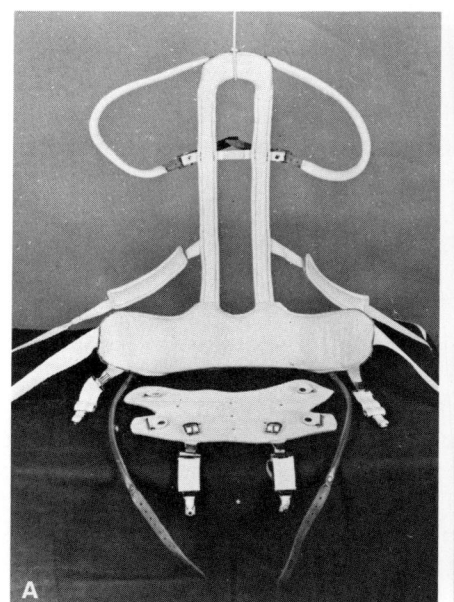

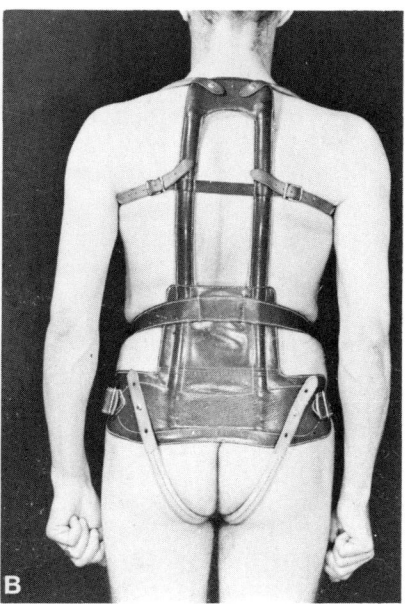

Fig. 116. A Jones brace before (a) and after application (b).

leather or vinyl. Two important parts of the structure are the padded shoulder straps which keep the patient against the posterior part, and the abdominal leather support which joins the rigid posterior part with two adjustable straps on either side. The abdominal portion lies between the anterior spines and is usually 5 to 7 in. (13 to 18 cm) deep. A narrow abdominal band is sometimes used, but the deeper one is more comfortable, especially for patients with weak abdominal muscles. Suspenders and groin straps are attached to lower front and side edges of the brace, these are necessary to keep the brace from sliding upwards.

Measurements. Ideally the patient should lie prone with a straight spine and shoulders slightly abducted. A posterior lay on cast is taken. First, an indelible pencil should be used to mark the seventh cervical vertebra, the posterior iliac spines and the sacral coccygeal junction. The skin is oiled, and sufficient plaster is applied to maintain the shape when it is set and lifted off the patient. The plaster shell gives the shape of the patient's back and also the length (the distance between the seventh cervical vertebra and the coccyx).

Three tape measurements are also required.

(1) The circumference of the pelvis at the level of the anterior spines.
(2) The distance between the anterior spines.
(3) The length of the shoulder straps. These are measured by placing the end of the tape measure on the centre of the spine at the level of the upper border of the scapular, taking it over the shoulder, under the axilla back to the centre of the spine at the level of the inferior angle of the scapular. The arm, of course, is slightly abducted.

The groin straps need not be measured as they are made 1 in. (2·5 cm) longer than the shoulder straps.

It is possible that the physical condition of the patient makes it impossible to lie him prone for long enough to take the cast. In these cases it is easier to obtain the shape and length of the spine by means of a length of malleable metal. The patient can lie on his side whilst the metal is shaped against the spine, the limits marked on the metal, which is then laid sideways on a strip of paper and an outline made against the metal. An alternative method if the patient is chair-bound, is to let them lean slightly forward, while the metal is shaped. The same tape measure measurements are required.

The Jones brace can be used for the patient who is to come off his plaster bed. The abdominal portion is removed from the posterior part, laid across the patient's abdomen, the patient is turned, the plaster bed removed, the brace applied to the patient's back, the fastenings adjusted at the sides, and the patient rolled over on to his back. When fitting the brace it should be seen that it fits closely o the spine from mid-dorsal region downwards. The upper end should be about two finger breadths space away from the spine to encourage extension of the spine. A brace should never push a patient forwards. An advantage of this appliance is that it leaves the whole chest free and so is often used for the elderly patient with osteoporosis and progressive flexion of the spine.

Taylor Brace

This spinal brace is very similar in construction to the Jones brace, the differences being that the posterior parallel bars end in the shoulder straps and that the abdominal portion is a rigid square one. It is consequently more suitable for the heavily built patient (Fig. 117). The measurements are the same as for the Jones brace.

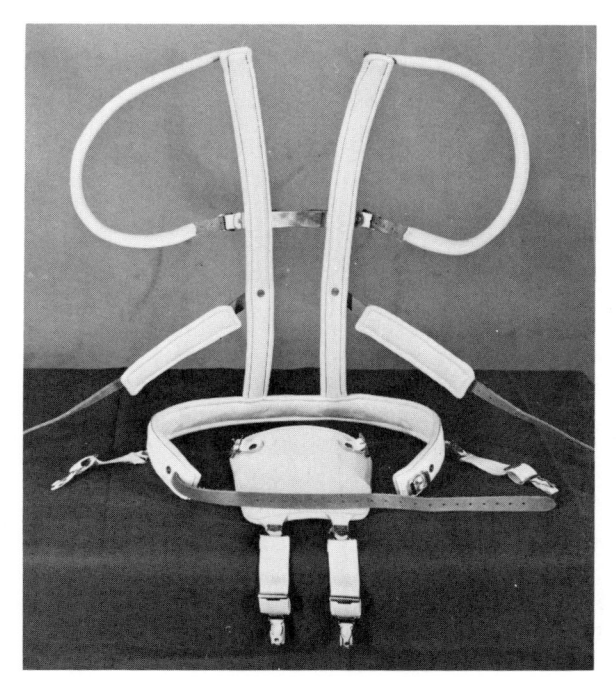

Fig. 117. A Taylor brace.

Milwaukee Brace

The Milwaukee brace (Fig. 118) is used for a mobile scoliosis in the growing child. It is designed to prevent, as far as possible, a spinal curvature from deteriorating. It does not cure, but by means of the distraction between the chin, occiput and the iliac crests keeps a

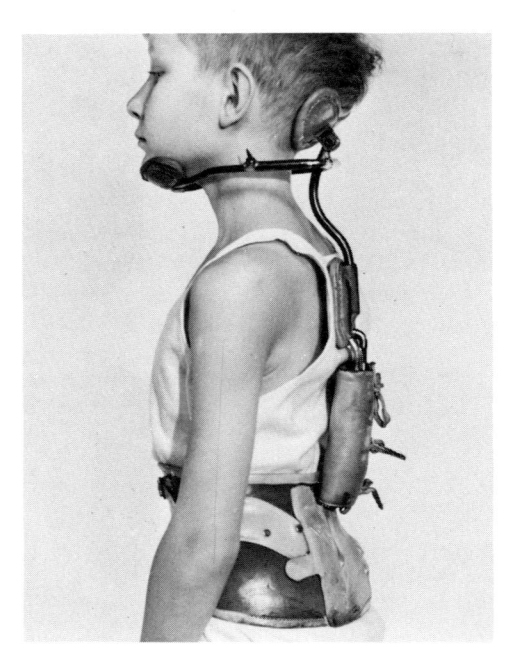

Fig. 118. A modified Milwaukee brace. Note the well-fitting chin and occiputal holds, and the pelvic support.

stretch on the spine throughout the growing years. The child with an ideopathic scoliosis or early severe polio may wear this splint throughout his childhood, until they are old enough for a fusion of the spine. The splint comprises a moulded leather pelvic belt with an internal sponge rubber bar which fits above the upper edge of the iliac crest. The middle posterior upper edge is joined to the turnbuckle which extends the length of the spine to the adjustable occiputal hold. The latter has tubular bars on either sides of the neck, ending in the chin piece. The side bars, with the chin attachment can be removed or changed. Sometimes an anterior turnbuckle is used which is attached to the chin piece above, and the pelvic band below. The fastenings of the pelvic band are central front in the first case, and on either side in the second case, and occassionally a sling is attached to the turnbuckles which supports the curve just below the maximum convexity. The turnbuckles are covered with a removable leather band to protect the skin. Two chin pieces are usually provided, as they easily become soiled.

The Milwaukee brace can also be used for the adult patient with ankylosing spondylitis. It prevents progressive flexion of the spine and relieves pain. It is usually worn for about one year.

Measurements. The measurements are taken by a plaster cast taken with the child suspended from the chin and occiput. The cast extends from the chin, occiput, neck, whole trunk and the whole pelvis. It is a difficult cast to take and an ordeal for the child. There should be two pieces of cast wire which are placed down one side of the patient, the top shorter length at the side of the neck, and the longer length below the axilla to the greater trochanter. The cast can then be removed from the opposite side. The cast is joined in the usual manner, filled, stripped and dried for 2 to 3 days in a hot cupboard. The cast should be inspected before being sent to the workshops. It is especially important to see that the iliac crests are well moulded during casting. It is generally advisable to build up the casts on the positive. This involves knocking two rows of small nails into the casts on the crest ridges. The nails should protrude in the centre by $\frac{3}{8}$ in. (9 mm) and are then graded at either end to $\frac{1}{8}$ in. (3 mm). These nail heads are covered with plaster cream, and so one is left with an exaggerated iliac crest. This makes it possible for the downward pressure to be exerted by the bars on the inside of the pelvic bands, over the tops of the iliac crests.

Application. The fitting of this brace is very important. It should be seen that:
(1) The pelvic band fits snugly.
(2) The turnbuckle does not come into contact with the patient (this is sometimes difficult when the deformity is severe).
(3) The chin and occipital holds are in the correct place, and at the correct angle. The attachment of the occipital plate to the turnbuckle is sometimes made so that the head can be rotated.
(4) The lateral neck pieces do not touch the neck on either side, this can be difficult if the upper curve is a high one.
(5) The turnbuckle is the correct length to obtain sufficient distraction.
(6) Finally it must be seen that the patient can just lift his chin off the chin piece. Half an inch should be sufficient play to allow for comfortable eating.

Maintenance. The patient should attend an Out-patient Clinic at bi-monthly intervals so that the splint can be checked as the child grows. The child should never be able to lift his chin over the edge of the chin piece—the stretch of the spine will be lost if he can do so—therefore the turnbuckle should be lengthened with the small key provided, until he has to hold his head up to avoid pressure under the chin. When the turnbuckle has been screwed to its full length a new one can be fixed into its place. The chin pieces can be re-covered when necessary. The pelvic band can be adjusted or relined when necessary. The child should, if possible, be supervised by a dentist. Changes which can occur in the jaws due to continuous pressure over a long period can be mitigated by the use of specially made teeth braces.

Blount Brace

The Blount brace (Fig. 119) is also a distraction splint for the patient with the mobile scoliosis. It is a more rigid splint than the

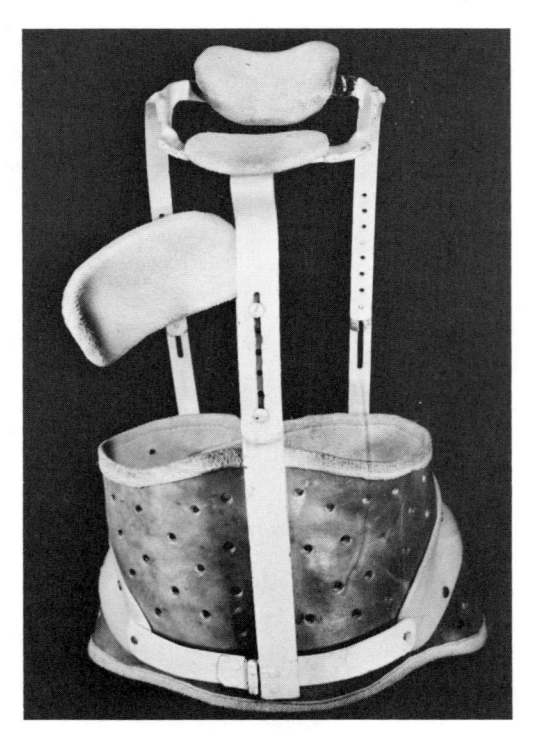

Fig. 119. A Blount brace.

Milwaukee brace and so exerts a more positive distraction. The same moulded leather pelvic band is used with the inner downward pressure on the iliac crests. There are two anterior and posterior metal bars connecting the pelvic bands with the chin and occiput. These bars are made with vertical sliding adjustments. The opening is at the back, and the occipital hold has a wing nut at one side and the apparatus opens by swivelling at either end of the chin piece, so that the splint opens at the back and is applied from the front. The chin piece is flat and does not exert the same external pressure on the lower mandible as the moulded chin piece of the Milwaukee brace. It is possible to make the pelvic band, chin and occiputal pieces of Formasplint, polypropelane or polythene. A throat hold instead of a chin piece is beginning to be used as this prevents the damaging pressure to the jaws. It is not as uncomfortable as one imagines.

Halo Pelvic Traction

This apparatus (Fig. 120) provides distraction of the spine between the head and pelvis by external traction and fixation. It was used initially for patients with severe tubercular kyphosis, but it is also used for severe scoliosis before fusion. The patient is able to walk about with it on unless the spine is unstable. Care has to be taken if there is paralysis of the hip muscles when excessive traction may cause dislocation of the hips.

Description. The apparatus is composed of four extension bars attached at the top to the halo and the bottom to the pelvic hoop. There is an adjustable pressure pad which is attached to the two posterior extension bars. This can be positioned over the maximum convexity of the curve. The extension bars are made of 9·5-mm stainless steel with 1-mm threads, and the bars may be bent to allow arm movement and accommodate rib bulge or kyphosis. The halo has four Allen screws to fix the upper ends of the extension bars. The pelvic hoop has four attachments through which the lower ends of the bars pass, these are kept in place by locking nuts above and below each bar attachment. When the nuts are screwed down, the length of the extension bars is increased. This lengthening provides gradual correction of the deformity. The distraction is begun after the splint has been worn for a few days, then the lengthening is begun by screwing the bars down 2 mm each day. The adjustable metal padded pressure pad is gradually screwed against the promi-

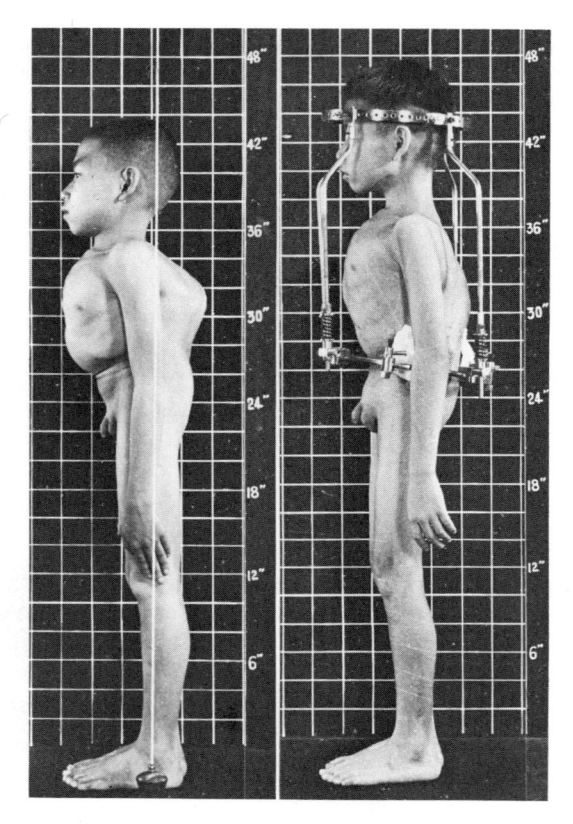

Fig. 120. Halo pelvic traction. Note the increase in height of the patient after application.

nence of the deformity. It is safest to insert a thick foam rubber disc between the spine and pressure pad.

Fitting. The patient should be anaesthetized by endotracheal anaesthesia. The pelvic pins are inserted through the wings of the ilium lateral to the anterior superior iliac spines, and emerge at the posterior iliac spines. The skull halo is fixed by drilling the skull for four threaded pins attached to the halo. The eyes should be well protected. The pelvic pins are fixed to the hoop and the extension bars adjusted. The use of this splint is justified in very severe deformities of the spine. Centres using the halo-pelvic splint usually keep a selection of different sized head and pelvic hoops. The four intervening bars are easily adjustable.

An improved halo pelvic traction is now used. The apparatus has the addition of springs at the bottom of each of the four extension bars and the force being applied to the spine can be measured. The anterior and posterior fusions are carried out when the full correction is obtained.

17

Collars

There are many types of collars depending on the seriousness of the condition and the speed at which the collar is required.

Soft Collars

These are the simplest and the most easily supplied collars. Adhesive molefoam can be used (Fig. 121). This material is supplied in sheets $\frac{1}{4}$ in. (6 mm) thick, 18 in. (90 cm) long and 8 in. (20 cm) deep. It is usually folded so that the adhesive side sticks to itself. The lower edge is shaped to accommodate the clavicles. The upper border is rounded by the fold. The deepest part of the folded strip lies in front of the chin. This controls or limits flexion of the head. Rotation is not controlled. The moleform is eased into a long stockinette tube which crosses over at the back and ties in front, and is easily applied by the patient. The folded moleform may also be cut

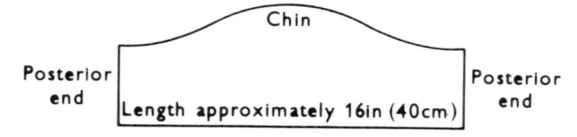

Fig. 121. Pattern for a soft collar made of adhesive moleform.

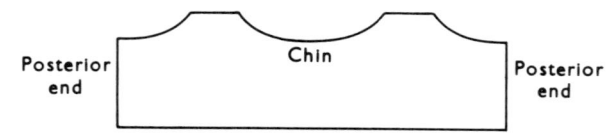

Fig. 122. Pattern for a soft collar with a cut to accommodate the chin.

to accommodate the chin and so further restrict movement (Fig. 122). Folded felt or sorbo rubber may be used instead of the moleform. Even cut cardboard well padded can be an alternative.

Plastazote Collars

These are very popular in departments where an oven is available. The operator stands behind the seated patient and applies the heated plastazote pattern and moulds it very quickly on to the patient. It is quickly trimmed to leave the ears free, and fastened with Velcro straps (see p. 40).

Polythene Collar

A plaster cast is required with the head held erect in the neutral position (see p. 34).

Moulded Leather Collar

This is an alternative to the polythene collar and is usually used when a collar has to be worn permanently or for a considerable time (Fig. 123). A cast, and fitting in 'the rough' are necessary.

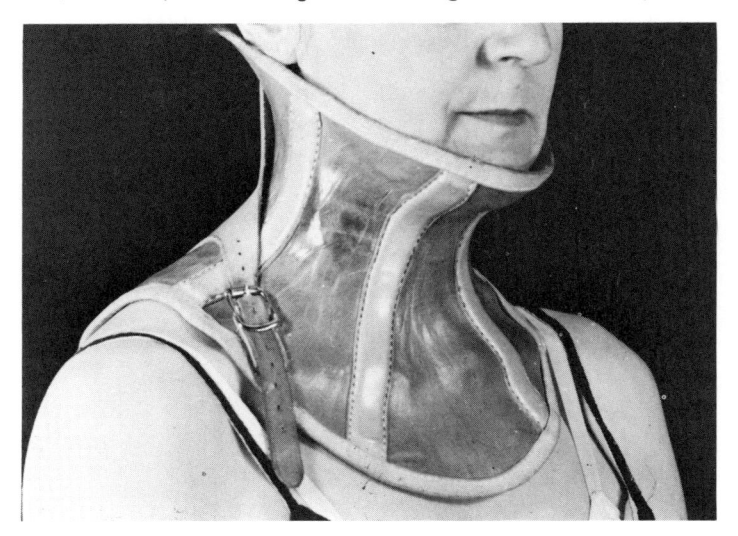

Fig. 123. Moulded leather collar.

Metal and Polythene Collar

A plaster cast is required for this combination. The polythene is used for the chin cup, occipital hold, breast plate and posterior plate. The intervening area being supported by two duralumin struts anteriorly and posteriorly. This ensures freedom in front of the neck. Naturally it takes longer to make.

Four Poster Collar

This is a collar which has padded polythene chin and occipital holds, as well as padded polythene breast and posterior plates (Fig. 124). The intervening area has four adjustable metal struts, two anterior and two posterior ones. These have turnbuckles to control the amount of flexion and extension required. There are additional webbing straps which should lie over each shoulder and under each arm.

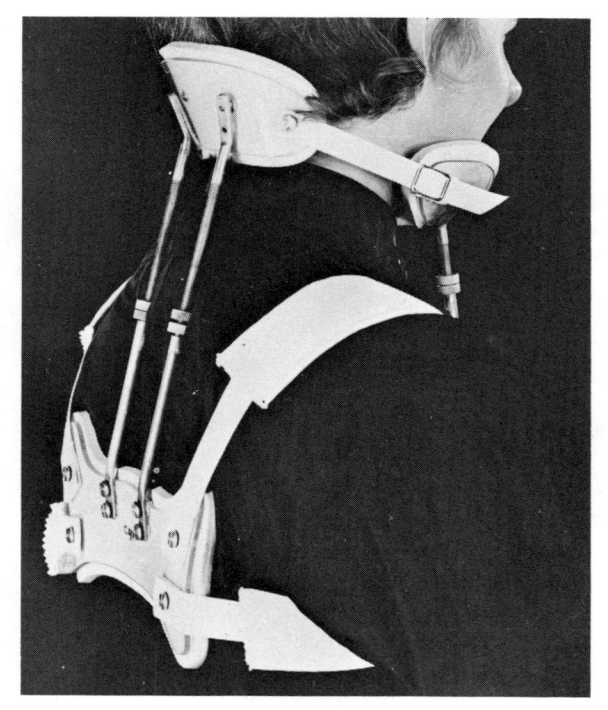

Fig. 124. Four-poster collar.

Thomas Type of Polythene Collar

This is a cervical collar with rounded soft rubber edges covered with leather or vinyl. The main part is made of perforated polythene and is fashioned by means of a wide Velcro fastening (Fig. 125). It is similar in shape to the soft collar.

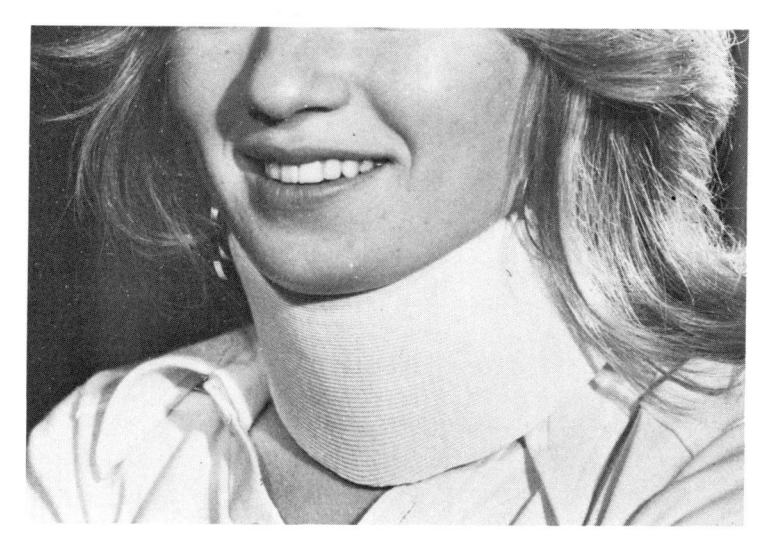

Fig. 125. Sorbo collar.

18

Surgical belts and corsets

Surgical belts and corsets are commonly used in the orthopaedic field. They are often used for the patient who has had a period in a plaster jacket or the elderly patient who is unsuitable for a plaster jacket but can tolerate a corset. They are usually made individually for the patient. There are many firms who specialize in these garments, and who employ fitters to measure and supply the corset.

In order to be able to give a patient a surgical corset straight away there are some made of elastic in a series of fixed sizes for adaptability. All corsets used for the patient with an orthopaedic condition should have at least one pair of posterior steels shaped to the patient's back. Correct alignment is very important both for the comfort and support of the back. The height of the corset in front determines the amount of flexion desired. When ordering a surgical corset the surgeon should state the amount of restriction required. Various additions and modifications can be carried out individually.

SACRO-ILIAC BELTS

When the support extends from the waist downwards, it is usually known as a surgical belt. Sacro-iliac belts (Fig. 126) are a very useful support for the man with a heavy manual job who has suffered a disc lesion. Posterior steels are incorporated, and are made so that they can be removed for washing purposes. There is usually an over-riding pelvic band which is wide at the back and narrows to the front. The belt fastens in front with straps and buckles and has groin straps or suspenders to prevent it slipping upwards. The material used for the

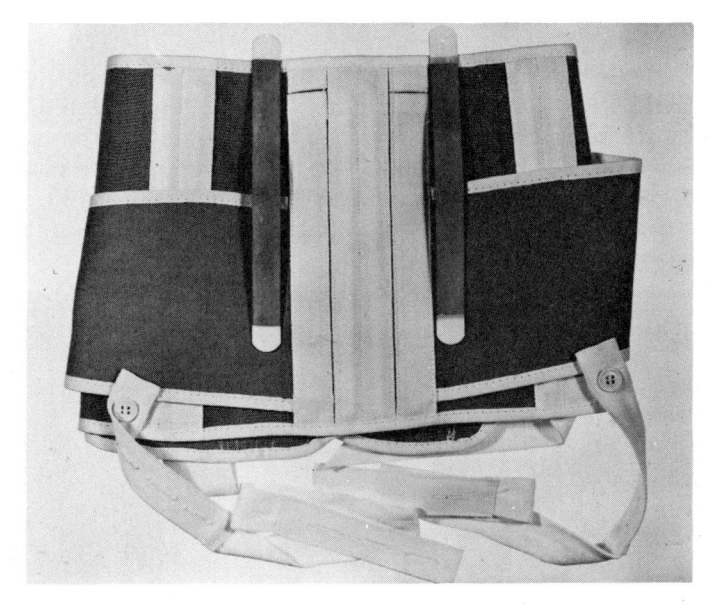

Fig. 126. Sacro-iliac belt, showing steels which have been removed from their sockets. Note the groin straps to prevent the belt from riding upwards.

male patient is strong contil and is usually grey or white. Female patients have a choice of flesh colour or white.

Measurements. The measurements for sacro-iliac belt are as follows:
(1) Circumference of the waist.
(2) Circumference of the pelvis at the level of the anterior superior spines.
(3) Circumference of the pelvis at the same level as previously but the tape measure should be directed downwards to the pubis and then upwards to the previous level. This is important where the difference in the two circumferences will be noted when the abdomen is prominent.
(4) The depth from the waist to the pubis.
(5) The depth from the waist to the coccyx.

If the abdomen is very large, bilateral fastenings may be more comfortable. Four posterior steels can be used. Bones or stiffening are usually used anteriorally.

Lunt Sacral Belt

The Lunt belt is a short belt of 6 to 7 in. (15 to 18 cm) in depth. It is made of strongly elasticated material with Velcro fastenings. The stiffeners are slipped into pockets at 3-in. (7·5-cm) intervals round the belt (Fig. 127). The stiffeners can be moulded to the patient and should fit snugly. The adjustable fasteners provide a 4-in. (10-cm) range of fixing. This is a useful belt to keep in a range of sizes for immediate fitting.

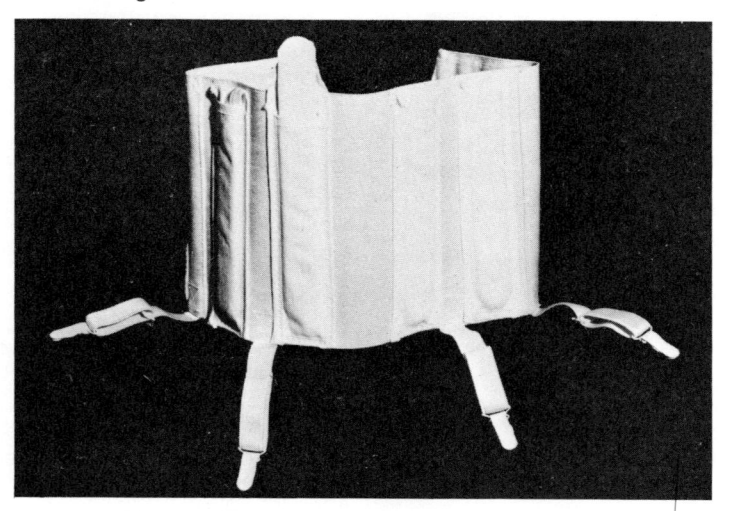

Fig. 127. Lunt sacral belt.

SURGICAL CORSETS

Surgical corsets on the whole represent the characteristics of the individual firms making them. In general, however, they all have shaped posterior steels, one or two pairs, extra pelvic bands and front buckles or lacing. They extend 4 in. (10 cm) above the waist to enclose the lower ribs at the top, to either the gluteal fold, or 3 to 4 in. (7·5 to 10 cm) below the gluteal fold. Bones or stiffeners are incorporated in the front of the corset.

Individual requirements for the patient may incorporate a supporting abdominal section for the stout patient, or elastic panels over the hips for the thin patient. Elastic gussets may be used at the top edge for the patient with prominent ribs.

High Corset with Shoulder Straps

It is sometimes necessary for the elderly patient with an arthritic or osteoporotic dorsal spine to wear a more extensive support. The fabric extends posteriorly to just below shoulder level and the steels to above the scapulae. The anterior top limit is just below the breasts. It is most satisfactory to incorporate shoulder straps which cross over posteriorly and fasten at the front sides. This ensures the patient being kept back in contact with the steels, although not all patients tolerate the shoulder straps.

Measurements. The measurements involve a series of circumferences with a firm tape measure. The depth measurement should be from the top edge to the waist and from the waist to the lower edge. Extra depth measurements should be taken if the abdomen is prominent.

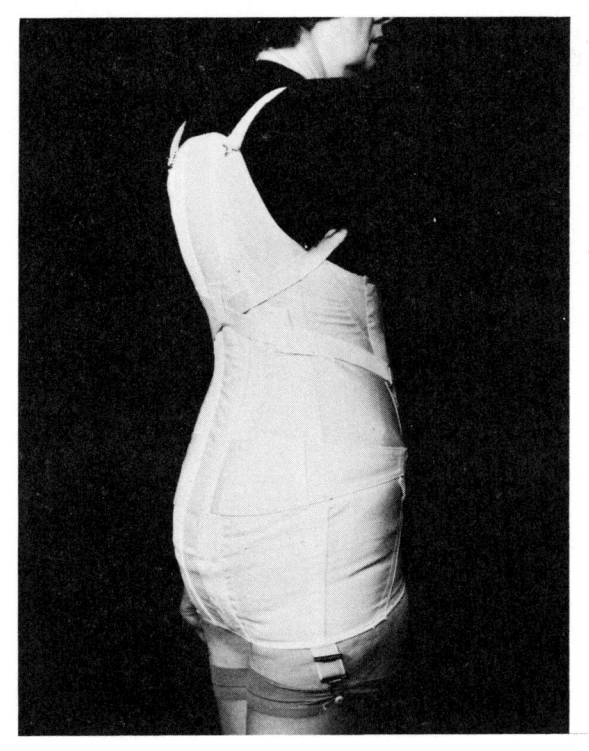

Fig. 128. High Spencer corset showing shoulder straps and well-shaped posterior steels.

Circumferences are taken of the trunk at roughly 4 in. (10 cm) intervening spaces, with length measurements to link them together, for example:

(1) Circumference in. (10 cm) above the waist.
(2) Circumference at waist level.
(3) Circumference at the level of maximum abdomen.
(4) Circumference at the level of iliac crests.
(5) Circumference at the lower border or 3 to 4 in. (7·5 to 10 cm) below the previous measurement.
(6) Length from the top measurement to waist.
(7) Length from the waist to the next circumference.
(8) Length from the circumference at the iliac crest to the bottom border.
(9) Length from the top to the bottom at the rear.
(10) Length from the top to the maximum abdomen.
(11) Length from the mid-abdomen to the front lowest border.
(12) If there is no prominent abdomen, just the length in front from the top border to the bottom border.

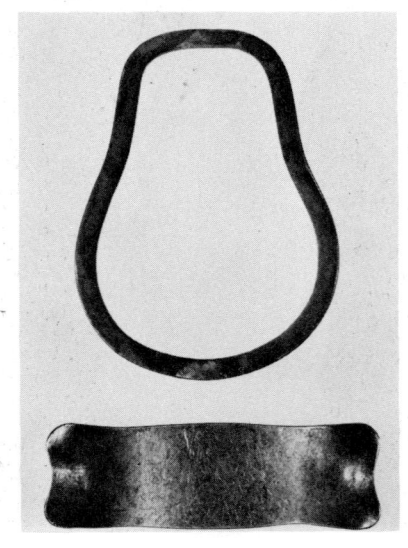

Fig. 129. J. B. Mennell plates. (Top) Posterior plate, and (bottom) anterior plate.

J. B. Mennell Plates

These anterior and posterior plates (Fig. 129) can be inserted into a belt or corset to give additional firm support. They are made from measurements taken by means of anterior and posterior lay on casts.

Measurements. *Anterior plate.* The patient lies supine and straight. The anterior superior iliac spines are marked with an indelible pencil. The abdomen is oiled and plaster applied with the anterior spines well moulded. When the plaster has set it is removed. The rectangular plate is made to lie between the anterior spines.

Posterior plate. The patient lies prone and straight. The posterior iliac spines and sacral–coccygeal junction are marked with an indelible pencil—the skin oiled, and the plaster applied from the waist to the coccyx across the back and lifted off when set.

These two plaster shells give the required shape for the plates which are sewn in position on the belt or corset, and they are covered with chamois leather.

19
Crutches and walking aids

CRUTCHES

Stocks of crutches, both elbow and axillary are usually kept in Casualty or Orthopaedic Centres.

Axillary Crutches

Axillary crutches are the most often used for patients who need them for a short period. If used for too long they may cause undue pressure in the axillae with resulting radial paralysis of the forearm. The upper edge should, therefore, be padded with leather, or just a leather sling may be used. The end should have a tightly fitting crutch rubber of the non-slip variety. It is more economical to have the lower end adjustable, and fixed with wing nuts. The hand grip may also be adjustable.

Measurements. One measurement only is required, that is the length from the axilla to the plantar surface of the heel with 1 in. (2·5 cm) added for the approximate height of the patient's heel. The patient should lie straight with the legs together for the measurement.

Elbow Crutches

These are usually made of chromium plated steel tubing and are designed to withstand rough treatment. The armbands are covered with leather or plastic material and the hand grips contoured to fit the hands. They may be made in junior and adult sizes, or they may be made adjustable. The length can be altered in the main stem by the lower tube sliding within the upper tube and being fixed with a steel peg which is sprung and can be inserted into one of a series of corresponding holes. The portion above the hand grip is not usually adjustable, but some firms will provide the extra adjustment.

Measurements. The patient should stand with the elbow flexed at about 130 degrees and the length measurement taken from the grip to the floor. An extra measurement may be taken from above the elbow to the grip.

Telcentric Elbow Crutch

The patient who depends entirely on crutches and yet needs to be able to use his hands at a sink or table finds this type of elbow crutch (Fig. 130) a great benefit. They are made of aluminium with adjustable ends and non-slip rubbers. The arm band has an automatic locking device to keep it in the upright position so that the patient can rest his weight on it. The locking device is released when the crutch is raised.

Elbow Crutch with Circular Arm Band

Some patients with strong arms and flail legs exert a great strain on the crutches. They find a completely circular band a help in that they can lean forward against the front of the band (see Fig. 131). Heavy duty chromium plated steel tubing should be used, and an extra measurement is required, namely, the circumference of the arm above the elbow.

The Arthritic Crutch

With this crutch (Fig. 132) the patient's weight is taken on the forearms. The main stem is fixed at right angles to the forearm support. On top of the forearm support is a short trough or gutter which has a wide Velcro fastening on which the forearm lies. A hand grip is fixed at the end of the forearm portion. It is usually in an upright position at an angle slightly greater than a right angle.

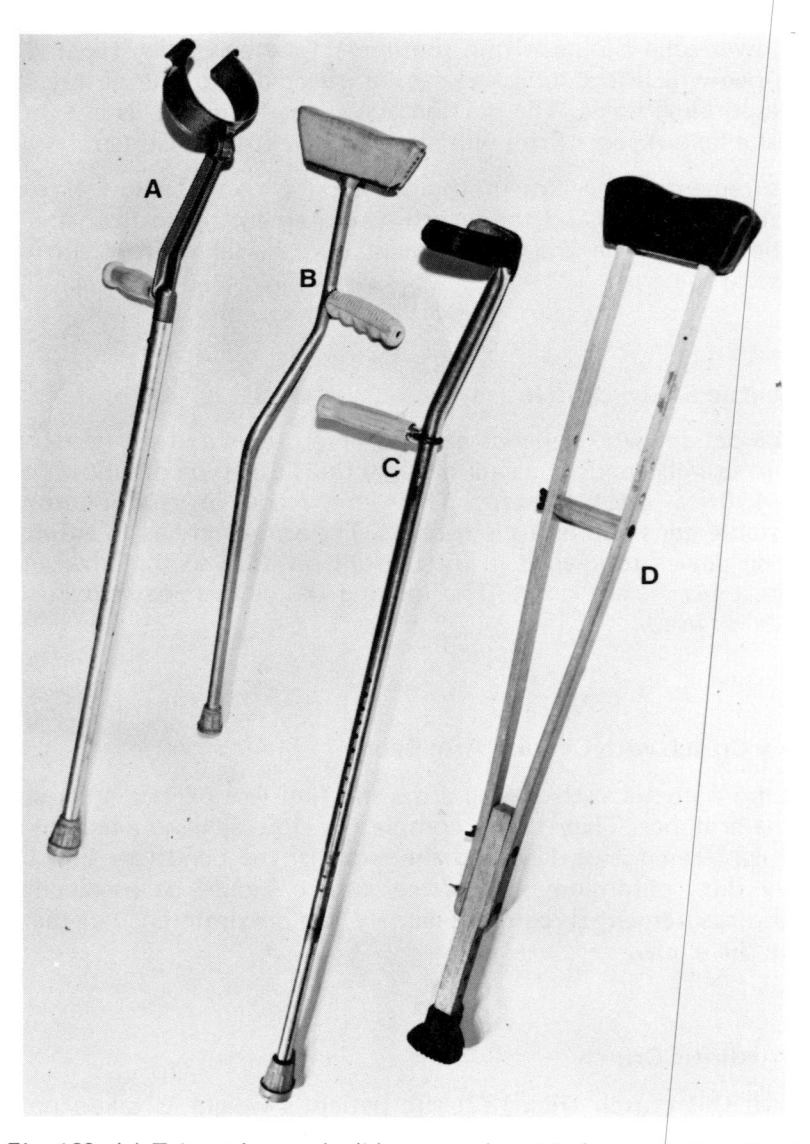

Fig. 130. (a) Telcentric crutch, (b) staggered crutch for use with an Harrison splint, (c) elbow crutch, and (d) axillary crutch.

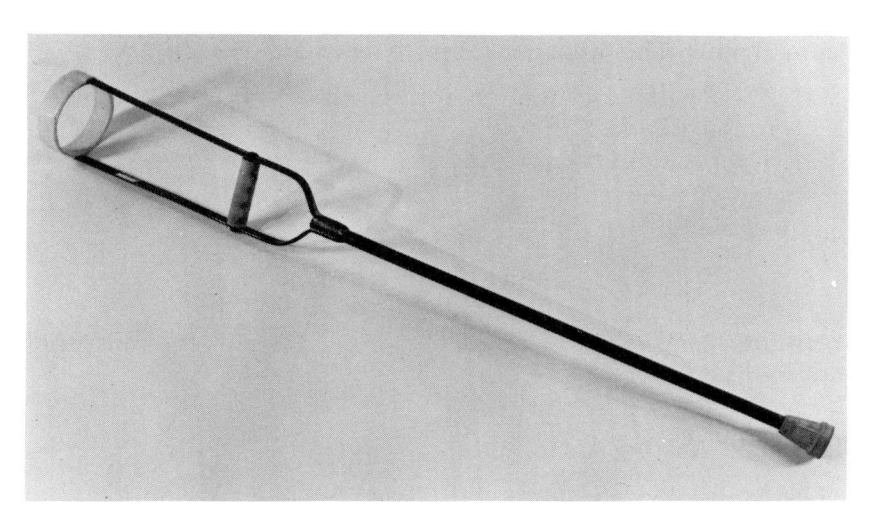

Fig. 131. Elbow crutch with circular arm band.

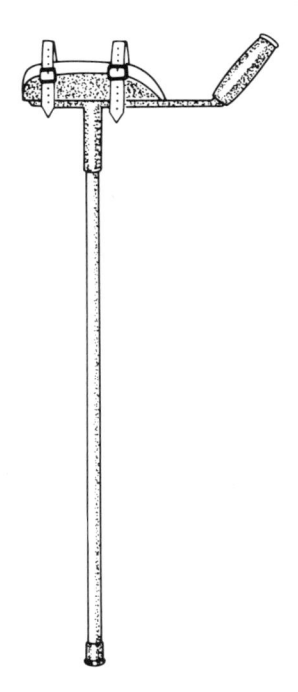

Fig. 132. The arthritic crutch.

177

Measurements. The following measurements are taken:

(1) The length from the forearm which should be at a right angle to the ground.
(2) The length of the forearm.
(3) The circumference of the forearm.

WALKING AIDS

There are many varieties of walking aids, a few of the most useful ones are listed below.

The Tripod Walking Aid

This is usually adjustable and is used for re-education in walking (Fig. 133A). It is made of chromium plated steel tubing and has three non-slip rubbers.

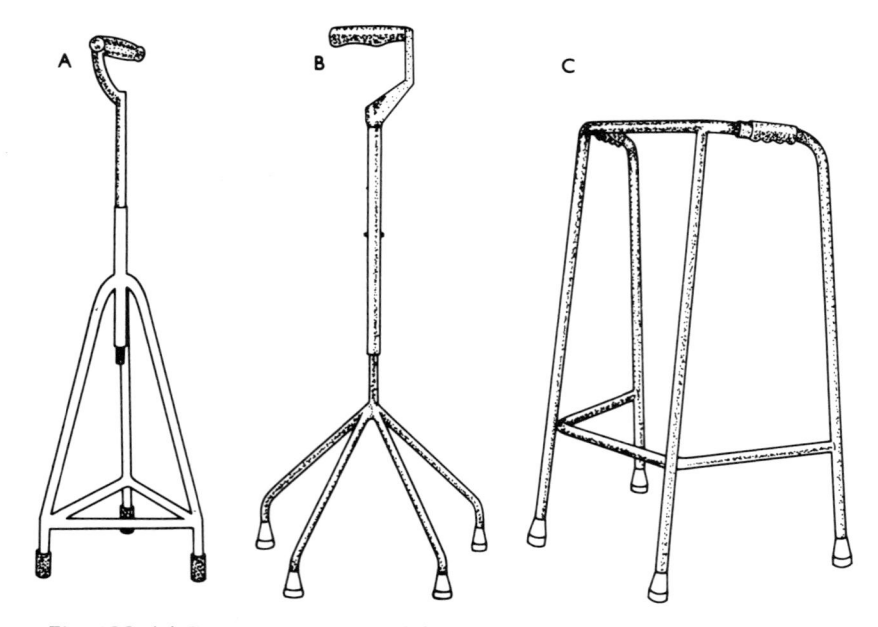

Fig. 133. (a) Tripod walking aid, (b) quadruped walking aid, and (c) a walking frame.

Quadruped Walking Aid

This is similar to the above, but has four stems joined to a larger central one and is designed to give maximum stability (Fig. 133B). It can be used singly or in pairs. The measurement for the tripod and quadruped aids is the length from the grip to the floor.

Walking Frames

These frames are quadruped in type but are so made that the patient stands within the frame (Fig. 133C). They can be used so that each side of the frame moves forward alternately or the whole frame moves forward.

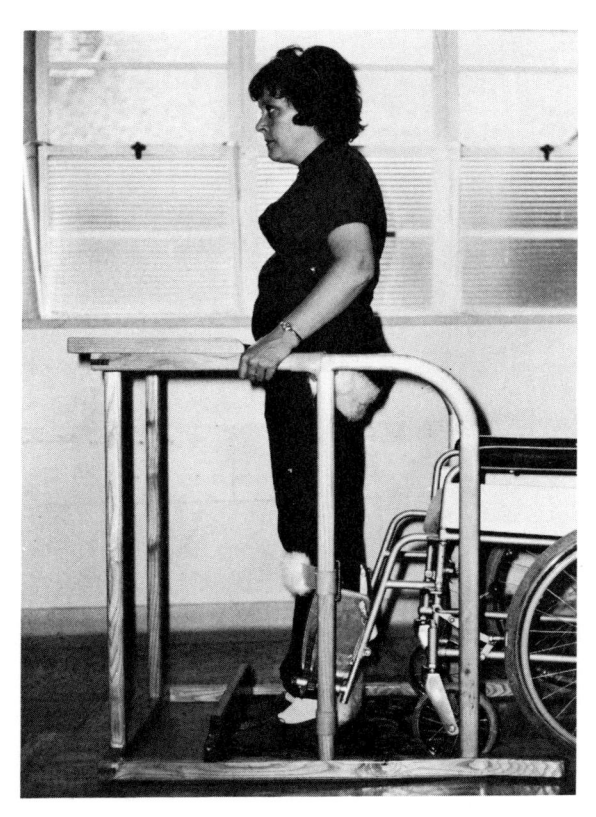

Fig. 134. The Oswestry standing frame.

Stair Climber Walking Aid

This is a quadruped type of aid with an extra pair of handles, which enables the frame to be tipped when climbing stairs. The lower handles should always be pointing up when it is in use for stairs. It has a specially strong basic frame.

The Oswestry Standing Frame

This standing frame (Fig. 134), designed originally, by Dr Nyquist of California, is used for the paraplegic patient. It enables the patient to stand without the assistance of calipers. The patient, with the aid of sheepskin straps placed behind the pelvis, in front of and below

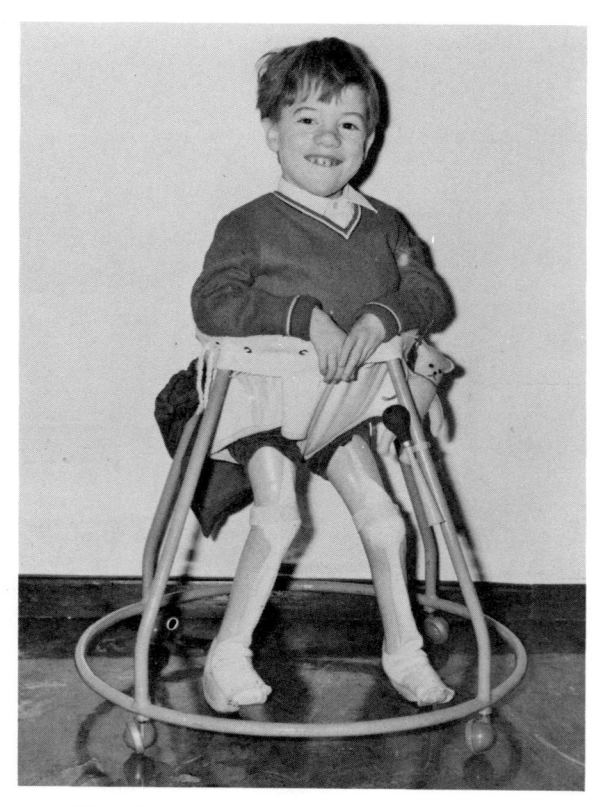

Fig. 135. The lobster pot walking machine.

the knees, and behind the ankles, is able to haul herself out of a wheel chair. The framework can be made of wood or metal.

The Lobster Pot Walking Machine

This is a circular framework run on ball bearing wheels, and has suspended in the middle, a canvas bag with two leg apertures. A smaller circular ring is fixed above the basic ring (Fig. 135). The baby is supported within the canvas sling and holds on to the upper ring. It is an excellent means of holding the later walker erect, at the same time allowing the legs to feel the floor. The machine moves easily but takes up a fair amount of room. It is useful for spastic children. It should not be used after the child can walk as it can encourage bad habits. The canvas slings can be changed and washed. The measurement necessary is the length from the grip to the floor, the rest of the machine being made in proportion to this measurement.

Babies Hip Spica Trolley

The baby encased in a hip spica after rotation osteotomies of the hips is able to move around by means of this wooden platform. It is a

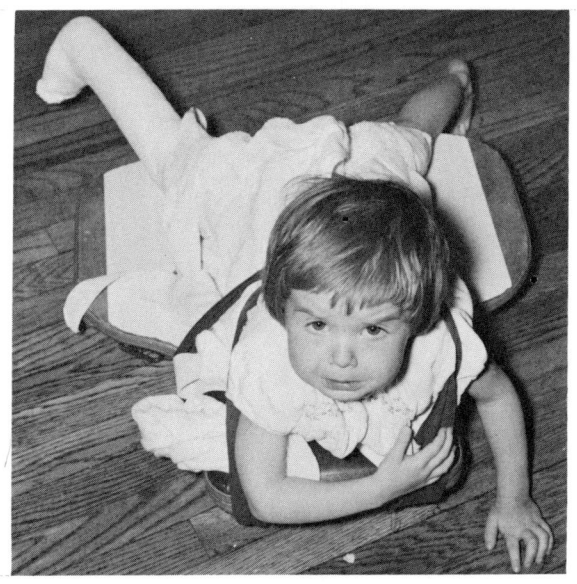

Fig. 136. Child lying prone on a hip spica trolley.

very simple means of locomotion, being a piece of hardboard on small wheels (Fig. 136). The platform is wide enough from the waist downwards to support the abducted legs. It is narrower from the waist upwards to enable the child to use the arms and to anchor the waist and shoulder straps. The child lies prone and is able to play with other children on the floor.

20
Bed appliances

Appliances for the patient confined to bed are designed only for bed treatment.

Pelvic and Head Traction

Many patients are treated for slipped discs by bed traction. Traction can be applied simultaneously at both the head and pelvis (Fig. 137). Sometimes only pelvic traction is applied, in which case

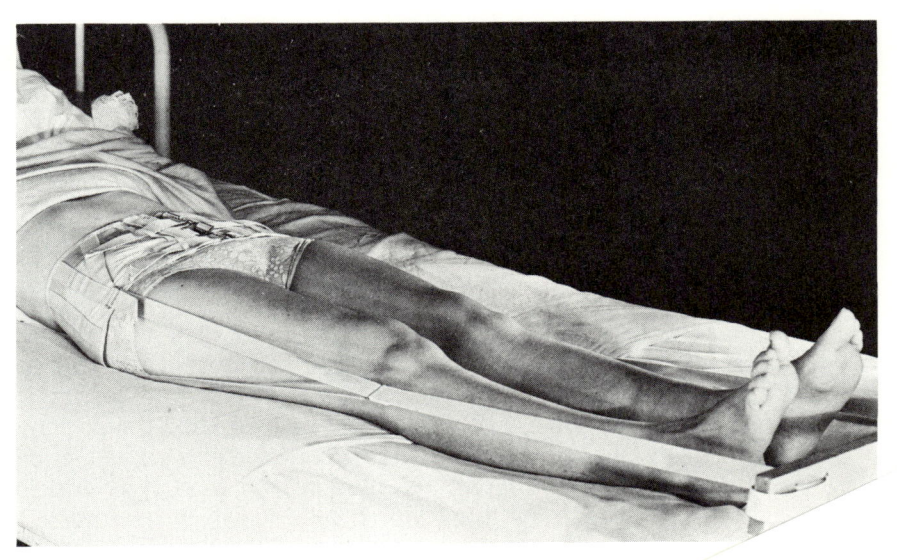

Fig. 137. Pelvic traction.

the foot end of the bed should be raised on blocks or an elevator. This prevents the patient from being pulled down the bed and it helps to increase the traction.

The Pelvic Traction Belt

The pelvic traction belt is made of canvas with central front fastenings and soft sections to grip and accommodate the iliac crests. There are lateral adjustable traction straps which are fastened at the end to a spreader. The extension cord passes through the centre of the spreader to a pulley, which is fixed at the end of the bed. The cord ends in weights of 8 to 14 lb. (3·5 to 6·3 kg).

Head Traction

The head traction apparatus is made of canvas bands, or strong washable contil. The posterior section can be made to cross over and so allow traction through flexion of the head. Self-locking buckles can be used at the sides to allow for size adjustment. The traction is maintained by pulley apparatus fitted to the head of the bed.

Spinal or Thomas' Straight Frame

This frame (Fig. 138) is used for nursing spinal conditions. The frame is made of mild steel 1 in. (2·5 cm) wide and ¼ in. (6 mm) thick. Two parallel bars are intersected by three horizontal bars. The top bars are known as the nipple bars, the middle bar, the Wingfield bar, and the lower bar, the pelvic bar. The nipple and pelvic bars can be hinged, and fastened with wing nuts. The Wingfield bar is placed 1 in. (2·5 cm) below the midpoint between the nipple and pelvic bars. The nipple bars are used to help keep the patient in position and also for an anchor for the shoulder straps to be fastened to. The Wingfield bar is used when the patient is first put out in the frame. The bars should be wrung upwards to push the saddle into the lumbar lordons of the spine. The pelvic bars help to keep the patient in position but are also used as an anchor for the groin straps. Lower down, the parallel bars abduct at the gluteal fold level. The knock knee bars are attached below this level. If a patient has to be nursed on a frame for a considerable period, the knees should be bandaged to the knock knee bars to prevent the onset of genu valgum. The two

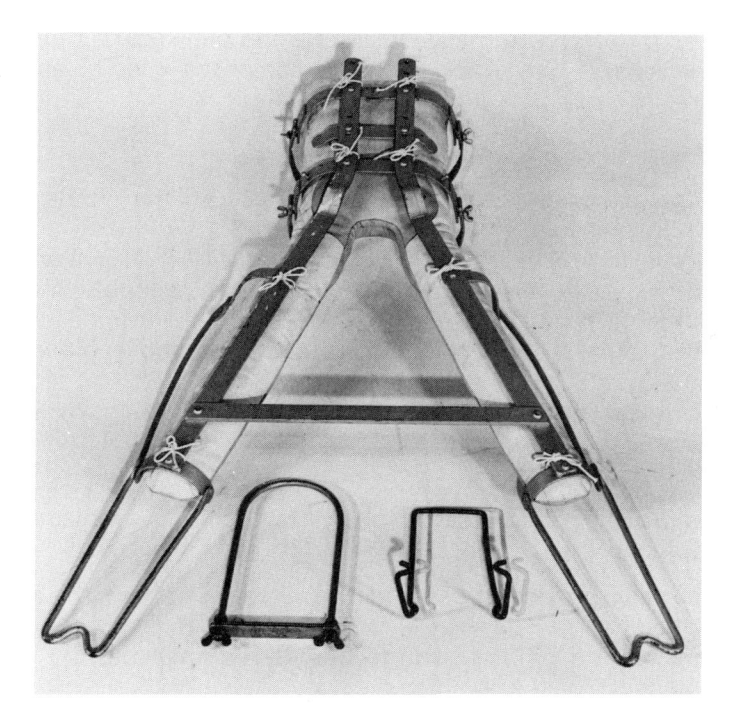

Fig. 138. Posterior view of the Thomas straight frame. This shows the nipple, Wingfield and pelvic bars. Note the two types of foot pieces.

bars are joined together at the bottom by a fixed abduction bar, and they end in the extension bows, the latter for the fastening of the skin extensions to maintain traction if required.

The spinal frame may have a detachable head piece fixed to help immobilize the upper dorsal and cervical spines. The extension bows have removable foot pieces fixed, to keep the bedclothes off the feet and to allow the feet to rest against them.

The Saddle

The metal framework is covered with a firm but soft saddle. It is filled with flock, covered anteriorly with basil leather and backed with canvas. The saddle can, of course, be replaced if necessary. Care should be taken to keep the saddle leather clean and soft. Some

185

centres use a frame with malleable nipple and pelvic bars, thus hinges are not necessary. The saddle may end above the knee or above the ankles.

Measurements. *The Frame.*

(1) Circumference of the chest at the level of the nipple line on full inspiration.
(2) Circumference of the pelvis at the level of the iliac crests.
(3) The length from either the shoulder level or nipple line to the gluteal fold.
(4) The length from the gluteal fold to just above the external malleolus.
(5) If a head piece is required, the length from the crown of the head to the shoulder level.
(6) The circumference of the head.

The saddle. The saddle need only be measured if a replacement is to be supplied.

(1) The length from the shoulder level to just above the external malleolus.
(2) The length from the groin to the internal malleolus.
(3) The width of the shoulders.

Application of the patient on the frame. The patient should be bathed and have had his hair washed. The frame should have its metal pieces covered with 1-in. strips of white cotton bandage. The patient is carefully lifted onto the frame, the coccyx on a level with the cleft in the saddle. Skin extensions are applied to the legs, and the Wingfield bar is adjusted if necessary. Groin straps are fixed to the pelvic bars and rear of the frame. The extensions are tied comfortably to the extension bows (true extension is not required on a spinal frame, in fact it need not be used, but it does help to keep the child in position).

Cotton shoulder straps are fastened to the rear of the nipple bars, brought over the shoulders, crossed, and tied to the ends of the nipple bars. The cotton slings should pass through leather cuffs which rest on the shoulders. The legs are bandaged with Kling cotton bandages directly over the extensions, and domette bandaging should finally be done to include the whole leg and leg portions of the frames. The nipple and pelvic bars are fastened.

The Abduction or Robert Jones Frame

This is similar in construction to the spinal frame except that the abduction bar is adjustable on one or both sides. Skin extensions are always used to obtain traction on the hip joints, and counter traction by means of one or two groin straps. The foot of the bed can be raised on a block or elevator. The measurements and application are the same as for the spinal frame.

The Frame for the Congenital Dislocated Hip

Though this frame looks a more complicated appliance than the abduction frame, it is basically the same (Fig. 139). It is designed to give gradual and complete abduction of the hips to an angle of 180 degrees. Consequently it is made with a curved abduction bar to obtain the full abduction. A straight bar could be used, but it would prove inconvenient, extending out on either side of the cot. The saddle has to be made in three parts to allow for full abduction, the trunk and two leg pieces being separate. The pelvic bars are used as an anchor for the cross pull which is necessary to keep the head of the femur in the acetabulum on abduction. The measurements and application are the same as those for the spinal frame.

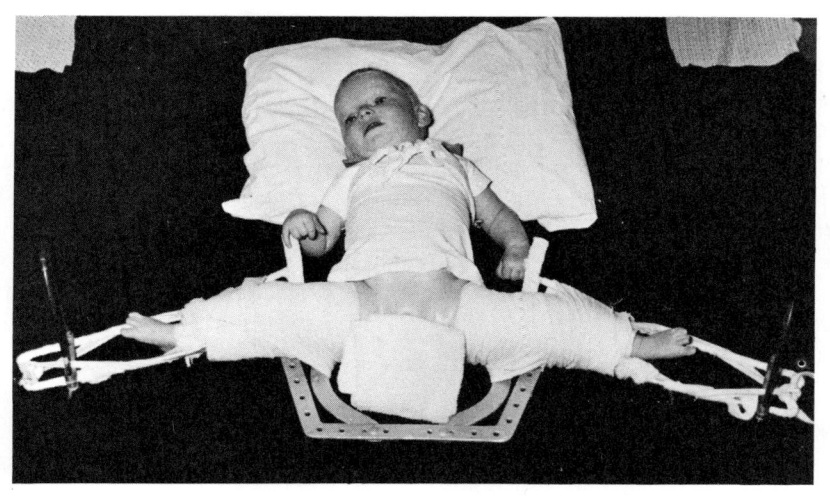

Fig. 139. Baby lying on a congenital dislocation of the hip frame. The cross pulls have been removed and the legs are fully abducted.

The Böhler-Braun Frame

This apparatus (Fig. 140) has been much modified since its inception. It can be used for resting a leg in the elevated position and for providing skeletal traction for some fractures of the femur or tibia. It is used after surgery of the lower leg or foot, as a method of elevation when pillows may be inserted under the leg on top of the splint. The whole apparatus can be folded flat for storage purposes.

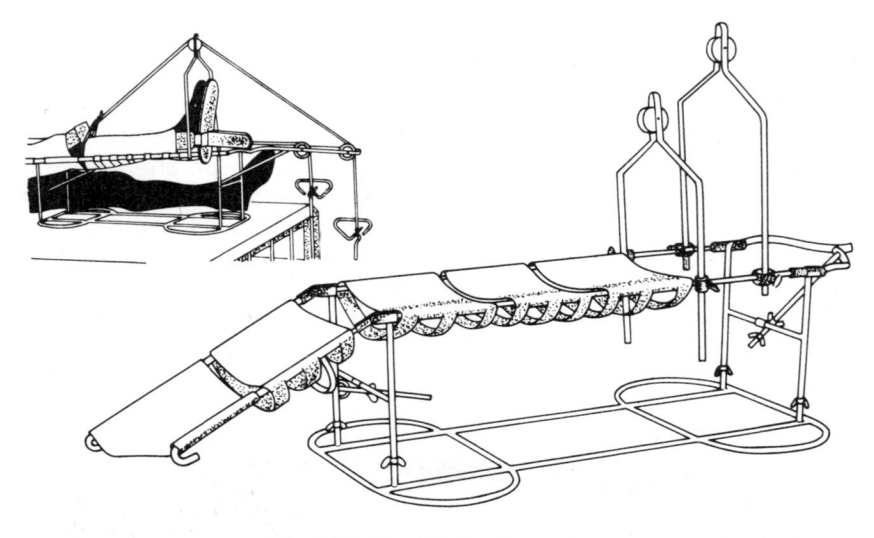

Fig. 140. The Böhler-Braun frame.

The frame is made of plated steel with detachable ends and sides. The femur end is adjustable in height and length, and the pulley arches are adjustable in length and width. A flannel bandage should be wound round the leg rests and fastened with safety pins, making sure that it is taut under the femur, but slacker under the tibia to avoid pressure on the calf muscles. A padded foot rest is usually incorporated to rest against.

Thomas Splint

The Thomas splint has been standard equipment in all casualty and orthopaedic departments for a long time. It is used for transferring patients with leg injuries from one centre to another, and also used as a bed splint combined with traction for treating hip and knee conditions. It is combined with accessories to obtain knee flexion, and correction of fractures. The ankle hitch can be used for transporting the patient.

Construction. The Thomas splint is made of two rigid double sheer steels (or, sometimes, chromium plated steel rods) which are attached at the top end to an ovoid ring made of the same material. The inner steel is shorter by 1 to $1\frac{1}{2}$ in. than the outer steel, thus the ovoid ring is tilted downwards on the inner side. The two steels are joined at the lower end by an upwards indentation for the ends of the extensions to be fastened. The back half of the ring is slightly larger than the front half to accommodate the thigh. It is therefore possible to determine whether the splint is for a left or right leg. The ring is padded with felt or foam rubber and covered with soft leather.

Measurements. The following measurements are taken:
(1) The circumference of the thigh at the highest possible level with the tape measure held firm and straight.
(2) The length from the ischial tuberosity to the plantar surface of the heel.

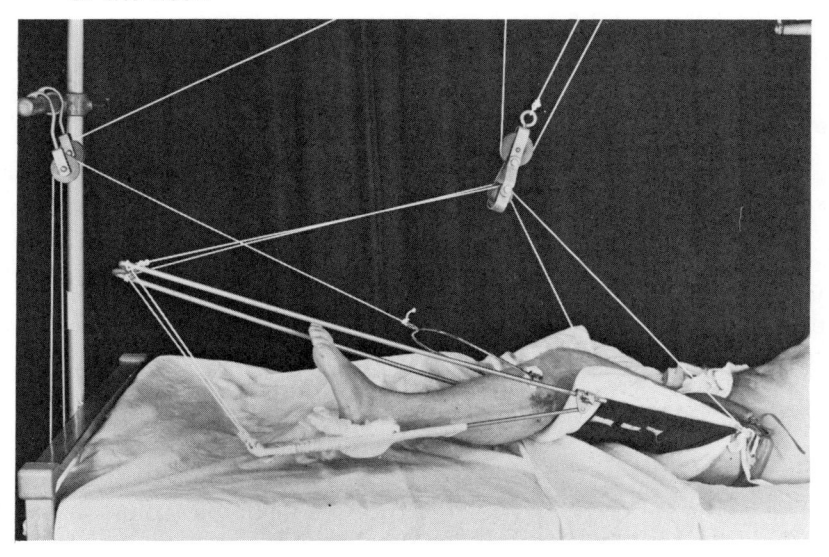

Fig. 141. A patient wearing the Thomas splint and Pearson's knee flexion piece.

Thomas Knee Bed Splint and Pearson's Knee Flexion Piece

The Thomas splint is used for immobilizing an infected or tubercular knee. In this case fixed traction is used. Skin extensions are applied to either side of the child's leg and fixed to the end of the splint. The ring should fit well round the thigh and push against the ischial tuberosity. The whole leg is then bandaged on to the splint, leaving the knee free. The ankles should be protected with felt or bandage, and a foot piece should be incorporated at the lower end for the foot to rest against. The patient can be lifted with the limb supported in the splint. It can also be raised from the bed by means of counter weights and pulleys fixed to an overhead beam, the cords being tied to the splint and separate from the traction weights.

Pearson's knee flexion piece can be fixed to the Thomas splint at knee joint level to allow flexion of the knee at the same time as permitting skin or skeletal traction. The lower leg rests on the knee flexion piece, whilst traction is obtained in a direct line with the femur by means of cord, weights and pulleys. The Pearson attachment is made of sheer steel or chromium plated steel with connections for attachment to the Thomas splint. The thumb screws are non-removable. The splints are usually made a standard length of 22 to 5 in. (56 to 63·5 cm).

Hodgen Splint

The Hodgen splint is similar in construction to the Thomas splint, excpet it has only half a ring. The application is the same, the half ring rests on top of the thigh, thus removing any pressure from the ischial tuberosity. Thomas pressure pads (slightly convex padded metal clamps fixed to a metal arch by means of a pressure screw) can be attached to the Thomas splint. This accessory can exert external pressure when required in some types of fractures of the femur.

The Alms Splint

The Alms splint (Fig. 142) is a modified Thomas splint in use at the Bristol Group of Hospitals. It consists of bilateral metal bars 1 in. (2·5 cm) wide and $\frac{1}{4}$ in. (6 mm) thick which fit the leg well. It incorporates a flat foot-piece which is adjustable. Behind the

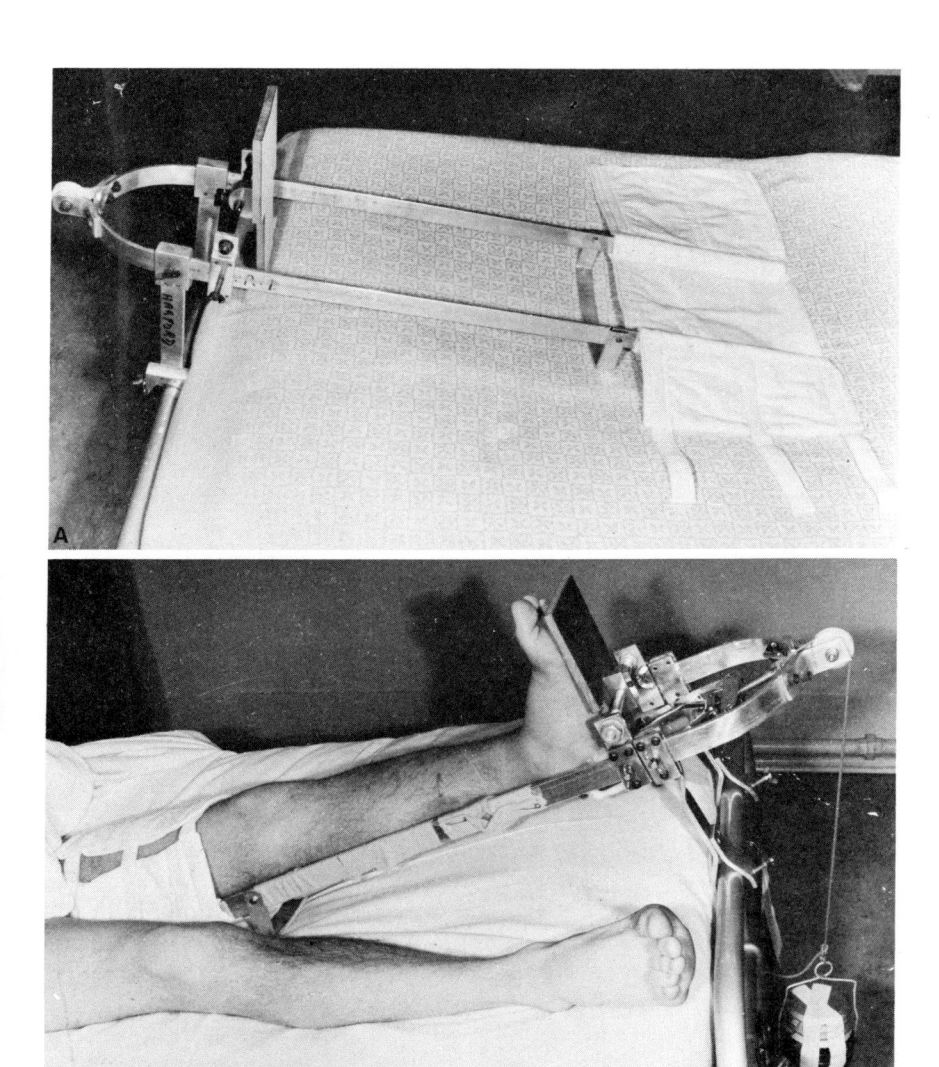

Fig. 142. The Alms splint before and after application.

foot-piece is a movable pulley mechanism which allows the necessary weights to be applied. The lower end is clamped to the bar at the bottom of the bed—it is used for fractures of the lower leg.

191

BED SPLINTS

Williams Splint

This bed splint (Fig. 143) is used during the first 7 to 10 days post-operative treatment after Charnley total hip replacement. It consists of two right-angled metal plates with sandals attached to the foot-plate portions. Below these foot-plates are four strong springs.

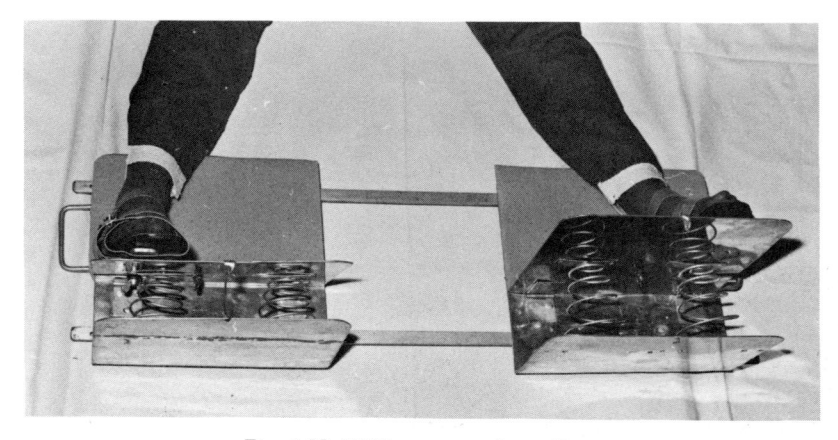

Fig. 143. Williams exercise splint.

The right-angled metal plates are attached to two horizontal bars which can be adjusted so that abduction of the hips can be obtained. Thus rotation of the hips can be achieved by the feet being placed within the sandals, independent abduction of the hips is possible, and the pedalling action against the resistance offered by the springs promotes good venous return which is important in the prevention of deep vein thrombosis.

Note: the calf area is completely free of pressure and that the handling of the patient for lifting and turning is made much easier.

The Cockin Exercise Splint

This bed splint (Fig. 144) is used for the patient during the first 10 days after the Charnley total hip replacement. It rests the leg and by means of the knee flexion piece, allows for active flexion and extension of the knee. There is no pressure round the groin. It is kept in position by means of overhead pulleys and Balken beam, 6 to 8 lb. (2·7 to 3·6 kg) being used at the head of the bed. The splint is primarily used to enable the patient to exercise the hip and knee himself. He can work the overhead pulley, thus being able to flex and abduct the hip.

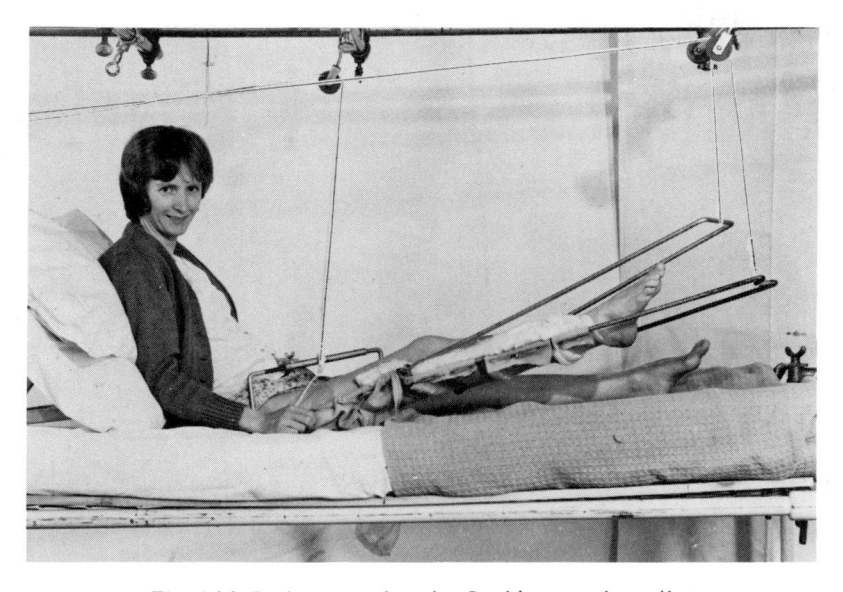

Fig. 144. Patient wearing the Cockin exercise splint.

Rolls Royce Bed

The Rolls Royce bed (Figs 145 and 146) provides a controlled traction for the patient with the congenital dislocated hip. The principle was first used by Professor Ivar Albik of Oslo and is now used at Oswestry. Rolls Royce have helped to design this special bed. The gentle traction holds the hips in abduction combined with medial rotation. Unlike the Oxford method, the process is a continuous one, and is not divided into separate phases of straight traction, abduction and cross pulleys. The child is able to move up or down the bed without diminishing the abduction. The rotation is kept at right angles to the limb. This is possible by the traction and

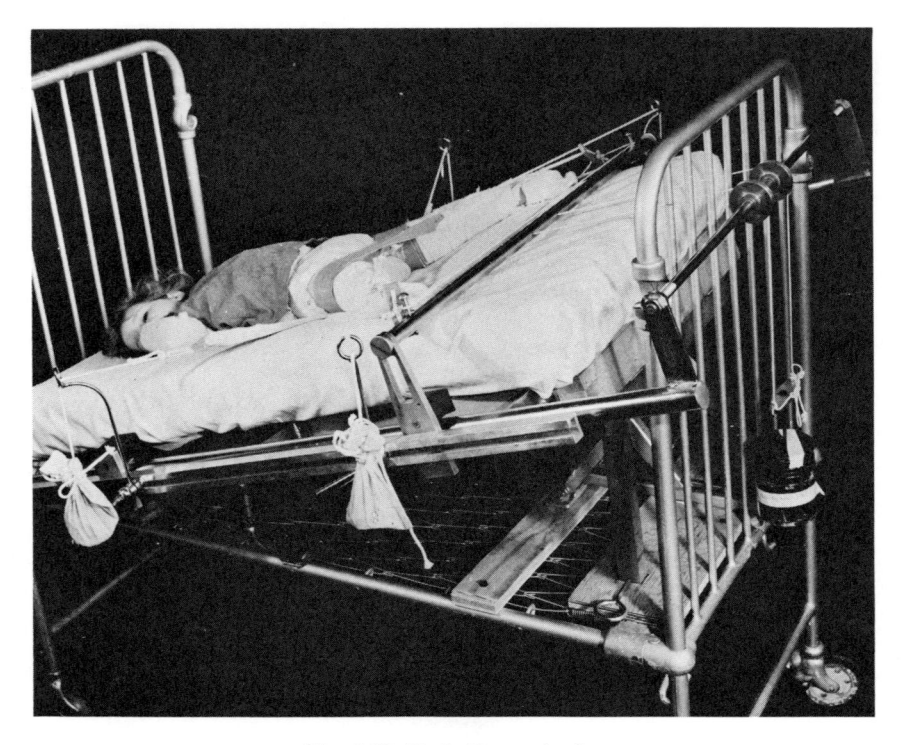

Fig. 145. Rolls Royce bed.

rotational pulls being fixed to the same free element which moves on nylon runners attached to the bed.

Procedure. The child lies supine, skin traction being applied in the straight position for a few days. Gradually increasing abduction is applied during the next 10 days and is then supplemented with internal rotational strapping. Longitudinal traction is built up to a maximum of 1 lb. (2 kg). The cross pull does not exceed 1 to 2 lb. (0·5 to 1 kg). Abduction is gradually increased to 30 degrees for each leg. The nurse is able to raise the end of the bed by a simple jack apparatus. The nurse must, first of all, attach weights to the cross bar and through this to the limbs—the amount of weight being sufficient to balance the child in any given degree of tilt of the bed. Once the child is balanced, additional weight is added for traction of the limb.

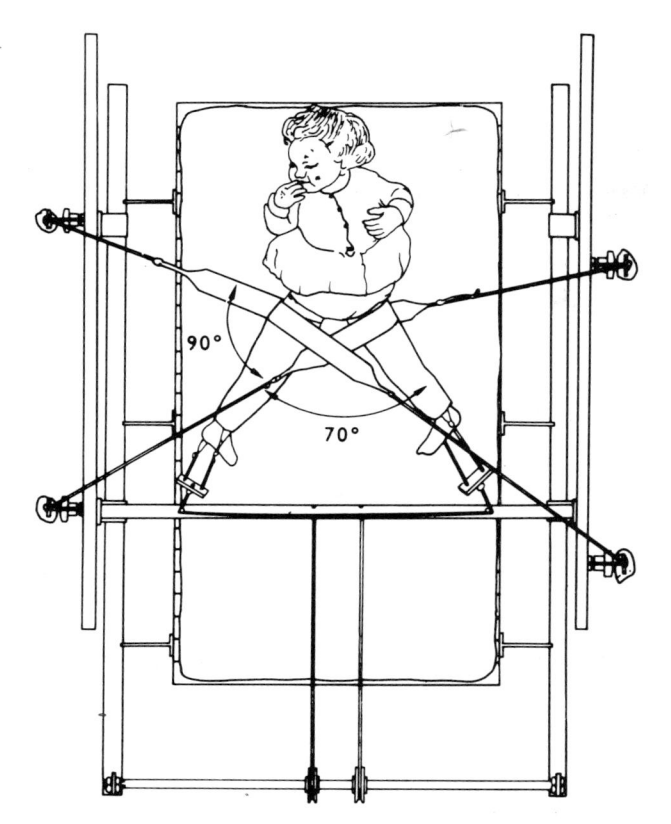

Fig. 146. Diagram illustrating the traction and rotation pulls of the Rolls Royce bed.

The weights usually start at 2 lb. (1 kg) and can go up to 8 lb. (3·5 kg). The rotational band weights are from $\frac{1}{2}$ to $1\frac{1}{2}$ lb. (0·23 to 0·78 kg).

Index

aeroplane splints   72-3
Alms splints   190-1
aluminium opponens splints   52
amputation stumps, plaster of Paris caps for   31
anti-pressure heel splints, polythene   34, 36
arch supports   *see* insoles and arch supports
arm abduction splints   72-4
arm slings   67-9
armchair splints   50-1

banana splints   133-5
band-topped calipers   79-81, 90-1
Barrow cruciform C.D.H. splints   111
Batchelor plasters   13
bed appliances
  Alms splints   190-1
  Böhler-Braun frames   188
  Cockin splints   192-3
  Hodgen splints   190
  pelvic and head traction   183-4
  Robert Jones frames   187
  Rolls-Royce beds   193-5
  Thomas splints   188-90
  Thomas straight frames   184-6
  Williams splints   192
below-knee irons
  double, with back check stops   123
  double, with Exeter coil   122-3
  double, with flat ends   119
  double, with front check stop   124-5
  double, with internal coil   122
  double, with round pegs   119
  inside, and outside T-strap   120
  inside, with flat end and outside T-strap   120
  outside, and inside T-strap   120-1
    with centre toe-raising spring   121-2
  outside, with flat end, inside T-strap, ankle joint and side spring   122
  moulded leather anklets   125
  shoe clasp ankle-foot orthosis   126-7
  Yates splints for dropped foot   126
belts   *see* surgical belts and corsets

Birmingham containment hip splints   104-6
Blount braces   160-1
Böhler-Braun frames   188
Böhler irons   15
boots for orthopaedic purposes   *see* foot appliances, boots and shoes
boots for wearing over walking plasters   15
boots on a bar   133-4
Bristol combined strapping and sole plate for club foot   135-6
broomstick plasters   16-8
Bryan Thomas lively splints   57-8
bucket-topped calipers   83-90
  fitting of   86-7
  non-weight-relieving   87-90
  plaster of Paris casts for   84-6

calipers   75-6
  band-topped   79-81
  bucket-topped   83-90
  Carshalton   97-9
  double, with pelvic band   93
    and hip joints with gluteal elastic straps   99-102
  full leg, with mobile jacket   98-9
  patten-ended   81-3
  ring   76-9
  Sheffield   96
  Stanmore   91-3
Camp Steeper radial splints   58
Carshalton calipers   97-9
cervical collars
  four-poster   166
  metal and polythene   166
  moulded leather   165
  Plastazote   40-1, 165
  plaster of Paris   10-1
  polythene   34-5, 165-7
  soft   164-5, 167
  Thomas   167
Chinese heels   15, 18
clavicle splints   70-1
club foot, appliances for   *see* congenital foot deformity, appliances for
cock-up splints, metal   65-6
Cockin exercise splints   192-3

197

collar and cuff slings 67-8
collars *see* cervical collars
Colles plasters 7-8
congenital dislocation of hip, appliances for
　　Barlow cruciform splints 111
　　Craig adjustable splints 111-3
　　Denis Browne splints 110-1
　　double nappies 113
　　Forrester-Brown splints 109
　　frames 187
　　plasters 13
　　Rolls-Royce beds 193-5
　　Von Rosen splints 109-10
congenital foot deformity, appliances for
　　banana splints 133-5
　　boots on a bar 133-4
　　Bristol combined strapping and sole plate 135-6
　　Denis Browne splints 128-31
　　hobble splints 131-2
　　Kites plasters 21-2
　　Robert Jones shoes 132
　　strapping correction 128
　　surgical footwear 146-9
corsets *see* surgical belts and corsets
Craig adjustable splints 111-3
cricket splints 48-50
crutches and walking aids
　　arthritis crutches 175, 178
　　axillary crutches 174
　　elbow crutches 174-5
　　hip spica trolleys for babies 181-2
　　lobster pot walking machines 181
　　Oswestry standing frames 180-1
　　quadruped walking aids 179
　　stair climber walking aids 180
　　tripod walking aids 178
　　walking frames 179

Darvic splinting 44-5
Denis Browne C.D.H. splints 110-1
Denis Browne club foot splints 128-31
Dr Scholl's arch supports 140
domed insoles and arch supports 137, 138
double nappies for C.D.H. 113

elbow crutches 174
elbow, slings and splints for
　　moulded leather splints 68-70
　　plaster of Paris splints 8-9
　　slings 67-8

Fairbanks splints 73-4
finger and thumb splints
　　armchair 50-1
　　mallet 48-50
　　opponens 52-4
　　spider 54-5
　　Zimmer 50-1

Fisher braces 153
foot appliances, boots and shoes
　　insoles and arch supports 42-3, 137-40
　　shoe adaptations 141-6
　　surgical footwear 146-50
　　toe splints 140-1
　　see also congenital foot deformity, appliances for
forearm and wrist splints
　　cock-up, metal 65-6
　　Plastazote 41
　　plaster of Paris 7-8
　　polythene 36
　　Prenyl 44
Formasplint 44-5
Forrester-Brown C.D.H. splints 109
four-poster cervical collars 166
frog finger splints 48, 50
frog plasters 13
functional static and dynamic braces for rheumatoid hand 59-64

genu valgum and varum
　　heel wedges for 142
　　splints for 114-6
Girdlestone Mermaid splints 114-6
Glassona splinting material 38-9
glove opponens splints 54
Goldthwaite braces 152-3
gypsum bandages 2

hallux rigidus crooks 143
hallux valgus night splints 140-1
halo pelvic traction 161-3
hand and finger splints
　　finger and thumb 48-55
　　lively splints for the hand 55-9
　　Prenyl 43-4
　　rheumatoid braces 59-64
hanging plasters 9
Harrison splints 104-6
heel caps 140
heel splints, anti-pressure 34, 36
heel wedges and flares 142-3
hip spicas, plaster of Paris 12-3
hobble splints 131-2
Hodgen splints 190
home made plaster of Paris bandages 5
Howard Marsh knee cages 117-8
hyperextension spinal braces 153-4

insoles and arch supports
　　Dr Scholl's arch supports 140
　　domed insoles and arch supports 137, 138
　　moulded leather arch supports 138
　　Plastazote insoles 42-3, 139
　　Rose's insoles 137
　　Whitman's sole plates 139

jackets see spinal braces and jackets
Jewett braces 153-4
Jones braces 155-7

Kites plasters 21-2
knee splints
   Girdlestone Mermaid 114-6
   Howard Marsh 117-8
   moulded leather 116-7

lateral plaster of Paris beds 30-1
leather appliances, moulded 32
   anklets 125
   arch supports 138
   arm and elbow splints 68-70
   cervical collars 165
   hip splints for Perthe's disease 104-8
   jackets 33, 151-2
   knee supports 116-7
   opponens splints 54
leather opponens splints 52-4
leather radial splints 58-9
leg plasters 13-5
lively splints for the hand
   median nerve palsy 56
   radial nerve palsy 56-9
   ulnar nerve palsy 55-6
localizer plaster of Paris jackets 19-21
low plaster loss bandages 3
Lunt sacral belts 170

McKee braces 153
mallet finger splints 48-50
master template for static or dynamic hand splints 62-3
median nerve palsy splints 56
Mennell plates 172-3
metatarsal arch supports see insoles and arch supports
metatarsal bars 144
metatarsal straps 140
metatarsus varus
   boots on a bar for 133
   plates and reverse shoes for 143-4
Milwaukee braces 157-60
Minerva plaster of Paris jackets 16
Murk Jensen plaster of Paris beds 30-1

O'Connor extension boots 147-9
opponens splints 52-4
Oswestry moccasins 141-2
Oswestry standing frames 180-1

palmar splints 66
patten-ended calipers 81-3
patterns for plaster of Paris slabs 2-4
Pearson's knee flexion piece, used with Thomas splints 190
Perspex finger splints 48
Perthe's disease, appliances for
   Birmingham containment splints 104-6

Perthe's disease, appliances for (*continued*)
   moulded leather splints 106
   patten-ended calipers 81-3
   Petrie plasters 16-8
   polythene splints 104-6
   Snyder slings 103-4
Petrie plasters 16-8
Plastazote appliances
   cervical collars 40-1, 165
   forearm and wrist supports 41
   insoles 42-3, 139
   jackets 42, 43, 152
plaster boots 15
plaster of Paris appliances
   application, drying and padding 5-7
   Batchelor plasters 13
   Colles plasters 7-8
   elbow plasters 8-9
   frog plasters 13
   hanging plasters 9
   hip spicas 12-3
   Kites plasters 21-2
   leg plasters 13-5
   Petrie plasters 16-8
   scaphoid plasters 8
   shoulder spicas 9-10
plaster of Paris bandages
   constant immersion time 4
   gypsum 2
   home made 5
   low plaster loss 3
   setting time 4
plaster of Paris beds 27-31
   lateral 30-1
   Murk Jensen 30-1
plaster of Paris casts
   for appliances of moulded leather and synthetic materials 24-7, 46-7
   for bucket-topped calipers 84-6
plaster of Paris cervical collars 10-1
plaster of Paris, composition and setting 1-2
plaster of Paris jackets 11-2, 16, 18-21
   localizer 19-21
   Minerva 16
   Risser 18-9
plaster of Paris night splints 22-4, 39
plaster of Paris slabs, patterns for 2-4
plastic splinting materials see synthetic splinting materials
polypropylene and polythene splinting material 45-7
polythene appliances
   anti-pressure heel splints 34, 36
   cervical collars 34-5, 165-7
   finger splints 48-9
   flail leg splints 37-8
   forearm splints 36
   hip splints for Perthe's disease 104-6
   jackets 35,152
   knee supports 116-7

polythene appliances (*continued*)
    night splints   37
    opponens splints   53-4
Prenyl splinting material   43-4

radial nerve palsy splints   56-9
rheumatoid arthritics
    calipers for   90-1
    shoes for   149-50
rheumatoid hand, braces for   59-64
ring calipers   76-9
Risser plaster of Paris jackets   18-9
Robert Jones club foot shoes   132
Robert Jones frames   187
rocker heels   15
Rolls-Royce beds   193-5
Rose's insoles   137

S. Von Rosen C.D.H. splints   109-10
sacro-iliac belts   168-9
scaphoid plasters   8
Sheffield calipers and brace   96
shoe adaptations
    hallux rigidus crooks   143
    heel wedges and flares   142-3
    metatarsal bars   144
    Oswestry moccasins   141-2
    raises   144-6
    Thomas heels   143
    toe blocks for amputation of toes   141
    varus plates and reverse shoes   143-4
shoe clasp ankle-foot orthosis   126-7
shoes for orthopaedic purposes   *see* foot appliances, boot and shoes
shoulder spicas, plaster of Paris   9-10
shoulder splints   72-4
Shrewsbury splints   94-6
ski front surgical shoes   150
slings, arm and elbow   67-9
Snyder slings   103-4
space shoes   149-50
spider splints   54-5
spina bifida cystica, appliances for
    band-topped calipers   79-81
    Carshalton calipers   97-8
    double calipers with pelvic band, hip joints and gluteal elastic straps   99-102
    lower limb bracing with mobile jacket   98-9
    Sheffield calipers and brace   96
    Shrewsbury splints   94-6
spinal braces and jackets
    Blount braces   160-1
    Fisher braces   153
    Goldthwaite braces   152-3
    halo pelvic traction   161-3
    Jewett braces   153-4
    Jones braces   155-7

spinal braces and jackets (*continued*)
    McKee braces   153
    Milwaukee braces   157-60
    moulded leather jackets   33, 151-2
    Plastazote jackets   42, 43, 152
    plaster of Paris jackets   11, 16, 18-21
    polythene jackets   35, 152
    Taylor braces   157
spinal frames   184-6
spiral splints   106-8
splints   *see specific splint*
Stanmore concealed calipers   91-3
surgical belts and corsets
    corsets   170-2
    J.B. Mennell plates   172-3
    Lunt sacral belts   170
    sacro-iliac belts   168-9
surgical footwear   146-50
synthetic splinting materials
    Formasplint   44-5
    Glassona   38-9
    Perspex   48
    Plastazote   40-3
    polypropylene and polythene   45-7
    polythene   34-8
    Prenyl   43-4

talipes, appliances for   *see* congenital foot deformity, appliances for
Taylor braces   157
Thomas cervical collars   167
Thomas heels   143
Thomas splints for bed use   188-90
Thomas straight frames   184-6
Thomas walking splints   81-3
thoracobrachial spicas, plaster of Paris   9-10
thumb splints   *see* finger and thumb splints
toe splints   140-1
toes, amputation of, shoe blocks for   141

ulnar nerve palsy splints   55-6

Von Rosen C.D.H. splints   109-10

walking aids   *see* crutches and walking aids
walking heels   14-5, 18
walking plasters   13-5
webbing slings   68
Whitman's sole plates   139
Williams exercise splints   192
wrist splints   *see* forearm and wrist splints
wrist straps, leather   66

Yates splints for dropped foot   126

Zimmer finger splinting   50-1
Zimmer heels   15